High-resolution
Computed Tomography
of the Lungs
A Pattern Approach

High-resolution Computed Tomography of the Lungs
A Pattern Approach

Author
D Karthikeyan DMRD DNB
Chief Radiologist, Division of Computed Tomography and Body Imaging
Department of Imaging Sciences
KG Hospital and Postgraduate Institute
Coimbatore
Programme Director, Radeducation Pvt. Ltd., Coimbatore

Contributing Author
Deepa Chegu DMRD
Radiologist
Coimbatore

Hodder Arnold
A MEMBER OF THE HODDER HEADLINE GROUP

First published in India in 2004 by Jaypee Brothers, Medical Publishers (P) Ltd,
EMCA House, 23/23B Ansari Road, Daryaganj, New Delhi 110 002, India

First published in the United Kingdom in 2005 by Hodder Arnold,
an imprint of Hodder Education and a member of the Hodder Headline Group,
338 Euston Road, London NW1 3BH

http://www.hoddereducation.com

This UK edition distributed in the United States of America by
Oxford University Press Inc.,
198 Madison Avenue, New York, NY10016
Oxford is a registered trademark of Oxford University Press

Whilst the advice and information in this book are believed to be true and accurate at the date of going to press, neither the author[s] nor the publisher can accept any legal responsibility or liability for any errors or omissions that may be made. In particular (but without limiting the generality of the preceding disclaimer) every effort has been made to check drug dosages; however it is still possible that errors have been missed. Furthermore, dosage schedules are constantly being revised and new side-effects recognized. For these reasons the reader is strongly urged to consult the drug companies' printed instructions before administering any of the drugs recommended in this book.

British Library Cataloguing in Publication Data
A catalogue record for this book is available from the British Library

Library of Congress Cataloging-in-Publication Data
A catalog record for this book is available from the Library of Congress

ISBN-10 [normal]	0 340 90580 8
ISBN-13	978 0 340 90580 7

1 2 3 4 5 6 7 8 9 10

Typeset at   JPBMP typesetting unit
Printed at   Replika Press Pvt. Ltd. Kundli 131 028

What do you think about this book? Or any other Hodder Arnold title?
Please send your comments to www.hoddereducation.com

Preface

Lung diseases derive their designation from their anatomical location within the support structures of the lungs, or within the alveolar walls, or within the airways and air spaces of the lung. Detecting diffuse lung infiltrates on chest radiography is a common clinical problem. Many diverse pathological processes can cause diffuse lung disease. The presentation of these diseases can vary from acute to chronic and includes a wide array of radiological patterns that are optimally evaluated on high-resolution computed tomography of the chest.

Designed for easy reference, this thoroughly illustrated, portable handbook is a practical guide to performing and interpreting imaging studies of the chest. The first section reviews the fundamentals of high-resolution CT and presents chest CT protocols along with anatomy. The second section provides an overview of focal and diffuse lung disease.

The third section presents succinct, key facts about all commonly encountered pathologic entities, along with representative images and explanatory captions arranged in alphabetical order.

D Karthikeyan

Acknowledgements

This book would not have been possible without cooperation and support of a large number of people from KG Hospital.

Foremost thanks to my Chairman Dr G Bakthavatchalam MS, for his encouragement and support.

I thank Dr. Mahadevan and Dr Jaymohan Unnithan MD, Pulmonologists for their active support. Dr Kumar MD, Dr Kanth DNB, Dr Vijay DNB my colleagues and paramedical staff of the CT Scan and MRI Scan Department for their help.

Special thanks to my professor Dr I Kandhasamy, my teacher and staff at Barnard Institute of Radiology—my alma mater. My parents, Dr Balavenkat Subramaniam MD, Coimbatore, Dr Hariprasadchegu, Chennai for their guidance.

Contents

SECTION 1

CT Techniques and Anatomy 1

SECTION 2

Overview of Lung Diseases 17

SECTION 3

Cases
   1. Allergic Bronchopulmonary Aspergillosis 43
   2. Abscess 45
   3. Acinus 47
   4. Adenocarcinoma 49
   5. Air Trapping 50
   6. Architectural Distortion 51
   7. Aspergilloma 52
   8. Asthma 54
   9. Atelectasis 55
 10. Azygous Lobe Fissure 57
 11. Alveolar Proteinosis 58
 12. ARDS 59
 13. Aspiration 62
 14. Bronchiolitis 63
 15. Bronchiolectasis 65
 16. Broncholithiasis 66
 17. BP Fistula 67
 18. Bronchiectasis 68
 19. Bulla 71
 20. Bubble Lucencies 72
 21. Bronchoalveolar Carcinoma 73
 22. BOOP 74
 23. Bronchogenic Cyst 76
 24. Bronchial Atresia 78
 25. Cavity 79
 26. Conglomerate Mass 80
 27. Consolidation 81

28. Cyst 83

29. Compensatory Hyperinflation 84

30. Cystic Fibrosis 85

31. Chronic Eosinophilic Pneumonia 86

32. Cong. Lobar Emphysema 87

33. Congenital Cystic Adenomatoid Malformation 88

34. Drug-Induced Lung Disease 89

35. Emphysema 91

36. Embolism/Infarction 93

37. Endobronchial Obstruction 94

38. End-Stage Lung 95

39. Ewing's Tumor 96

40. Fungal Abscess 97

41. Fissural Fluid 98

42. Ground Glass Opacity 99

43. Honeycombing 100

44. Hypersensitive Pneumonitis 101

45. Pulmonary Hemorrhage 103

46. Hyperlucent Hemithorax 105

47. Lymphangioleiomyomatosis 106

48. Lymphangitic Carcinomatosis 107

49. Miliary Pattern 108

50. Mosaic Perfusion 109

51. Middle Lobe Syndrome 110

52. Mesothelioma 111

53. Neoplasia 112

54. Nodules 115

55. Obstructive Hyperinflation 116

56. Parenchymal Band-Linear 117

57. Pancoast Tumor 118

58. Pleural Calcification 120

59. Pleural Thickening 121

60. Pleural Effusion 122

61. Pneumatocele 123

62. Pneumothorax 124

63. Pleural Deposit 126

64. Pulmonary Contusion 127

65. Pulmonary Edema 128

66. Pneumocystis Carinii Pneumonia 129

67. Pulmonary Laceration 130

68. Pulmonary AV Malformation 131

69. Poland Syndrome 133

70. Rasmussen's Aneurysm 134

71. Reticular Pattern 135

72. Round Atelectasis 136

73. **Rheumatoid Lung** 137

74. **Radiation Pneumonitis** 138

75. **Silicosis** 139

76. **Sarcoidosis** 141

77. **Scleroderma** 143

78. **Secondaries** 144

79. **Septal Thickening** 146

80. **Subpleural Line** 147

81. **SPN** 148

82. **Sequestration** 152

83. **Tracheomegaly** 154

84. **Traction Bronchiectasis** 155

85. **Transbronchial Spread** 156

86. **Tuberculosis** 157

87. **Tree-in-Bud** 161

88. **Three Dimensional Rendering Techniques** 162

89. **Wegener's Granuloma** 164

90. **Sign in Thoracic CT** 166

91. **Air Crescent Sign** 167

92. **Drowned Lung Sign** 168

93. **Fallen Lung Sign** 169

94. **Gloved Finger Sign** 170

95. **Golden 'S' Sign** 171

96. **Halo Sign** 172

97. **Hampton's Hump Sign** 173

98. **CT Angiogram Sign** 174

99. **Signet-Ring Sign** 175

100. **Split Pleura Sign** 176

101. **Western-Mark Sign** 177

102. **Luftsichel Sign** 178

Appendix: Compilation of Useful Hints for Chest Imaging 179

Pullouts

1. *Approach to Ground Glass Opacity* 209
2. *Approach to Bronchiolar CT Patterns* 210
3. *Approach to Cystic and Cavitary Diseases* 212
4. *Approach to Eosinophilic Lung Disease: A Clinical Overview* 214
5. *Approach to Parenchymal Lung Diseases* 215
6. *Approach for Reticular Opacity* 216
7. *Approach for Nodules* 216

References 217

Index 219

Section 1

CT Techniques and Anatomy

Introduction

High-resolution CT (**HRCT**) is now regarded as an indispensable tool for the investigation of patients with suspected or known, Parenchymal lung disease. The cross-sectional perspectives and high spatial resolution make HRCT superior to other imaging modalities.

Parenchymal lung diseases include Airway disease, Air space disease and Interstitial diseases. The latter needs special attention since HRCT provides histospecific diagnosis in many cases.

Numerous studies have shown the basic superiority of HRCT over chest radiography in terms of improved detection of lung disease, provision of a specific diagnosis, and the identification of reversible disease.

INDICATIONS

INDICATIONS FOR HIGH-RESOLUTION CT
• To detect focal, diffuse lung disease in patients with normal or equivocal radiographic abnormalities.
• To narrow the differential diagnosis or make a specific diagnosis, in patients with obvious but nonspecific radiographic abnormalities.
• To guide the site of lung biopsy.
• To investigate patients presenting with hemoptysis.
• To assess the distribution of emphysema.
• To evaluate disease reversibility, particularly in patients with fibrosing lung disease

SCAN TECHNIQUE

To obtain an optimum HRCT few technical modifications are to be considered.

1. *Collimation:* Thinnest available collimation should be undertaken. This includes 1-2 mm collimation. Higher collimations (1 cm) reduces the ability of the scan to resolve small structures, however vessels can be followed more easily and differentiated from nodules, a disadvantage which can be overcome easily with experience.
2. *Reconstruction algorithm:* High spatial frequency or sharp algorithm is used, that is bone algorithm which reduces image smoothing and increases spatial resolution, making structures appear sharper.
3. *KV, mA and scan time:* In HRCT image noise is more apparent than with standard CT which appears as graininess or mottle, in addition using sharp reconstruction algorithm makes the noise more prominent. Most of this noise is quantum related, thus decreased by increased technique, that is kVp and mA or scan time. However as increasing scan time is not practicable and can lead to motion related artifacts the other two parameters are altered to reduce noise. The routine technique used for HRCT includes kVp of 120-140 and mA of 140-240. In recent years introduction of low dose HRCT using kVp of 120-140 and mA of 30 using 2 seconds scan time has proved to be an alternative approach. In a study performed by Zwirewich *et al* using 20 mA at 2 seconds scan time both conventional and low dose HRCT are equivalent for the demonstration of vessels, lobar and segmental bronchi, structures of the secondary pulmonary lobule and in characterizing the extent and distribution of reticular abnormalities, honeycomb cysts and thickened

interlobular septae. However low dose technique failed to demonstrate ground glass opacities in few of the cases. Low dose technique also proved to have more prominent linear streak artifacts. In conclusion, although conventional HRCT was more accurate than low dose HRCT this difference was not significant and both techniques provided similar anatomic information.

4. *Matrix size:* Largest available matrix size should be employed which is 512 × 512 for most commercial scanners including ours.
5. *Field of view and use of targeted reconstruction:* Field of view should be large enough to encompass the patient, that is 35 cm. Retrospective targeting image reconstruction to a single lung instead of the entire thorax, using a smaller field of view significantly reduces the image pixel size and this increases the spatial resolution.
6. *Image photography and window setting:* Even though there is no specific or ideal window setting for demonstration of lung anatomy in HRCT, it is important that at least one lung window setting be used consistently in all patients as to make the comparison easy and effective. The so-called lung window of −700 window mean/1000 HU window width for routine lung examination. This can be modified for visualization of specific lesions and targeted area approach.

Few alterations include:
- Window of −500 to −700/2000 HU could be employed for evaluation of pleuro-parenchymal abnormalities,
- Window of 30/350 HU can be employed for evaluation of mediastinum, and pleura
- Low window setting of −800 to −900 HU with narrow window width of 500 HU can be deployed for evaluation of emphysema as the lung tissue will appear gray and the emphysematous tissue will stand out.

In conclusion, window mean of -600 to −700 HU and window width of 1000 to 1500 HU are appropriate.

Interpretation of large images is much easier than smaller ones, we provide 9 images in one 14 x 17 film for lung window images and twelve on one film for mediastinum.

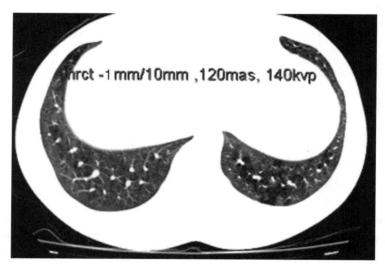

Fig. 1

ARTIFACTS ON HRCT

Streak and motion artifacts are two common types of artifacts seen on HRCT.

Streak artifacts arise from edges of sharply marginated, high contrast structures such as bronchial walls, ribs, vertebral bodies and seen mainly overlying the posterior lung, paralleling the pleural surface and posterior chest wall.

Motion artifacts or star artifacts are commonly invisible, particularly at a left lung base, adjacent to the heart due to cardiac pulsation.

SCAN PROTOCOLS

These include inspiratory levels, patient's position and scan spacing.

Scans should be done with breath held in full inspiration. However the use of expiratory CT has been reported in patients with emphysema, asthma, McLeods syndrome, cystic lung disease and in patients with variety of large and small airway obstruction. In normal subjects lung parenchyma increase uniformly in attenuation following expiration, but in presence of obstruction lung volume remains same and the lung parenchyma remains lucent.

Supine position is ideal for scanning, however in many normal subjects a "dependent density" or "subpleural lines" is seen in the dependent lung areas. These normal findings can mimic early lung fibrosis. This doubt can easily be overcome by taking prone scans. In case of lung pathology dependent density will persist whereas in normal subjects they disappear. In patients with evident lung disease and presence of dependent density, prone films are not required, as the pathology is the most likely cause.

HRCT for Interstitial Disease

Technique

Maximize spatial resolution
Thin collimation
High spatial freq algorithm
Additional Tech
Slab
Inspiration/expiration

Fig. 2.

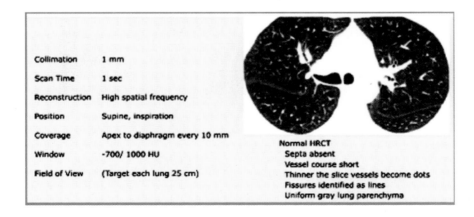

Collimation	1 mm
Scan Time	1 sec
Reconstruction	High spatial frequency
Position	Supine, inspiration
Coverage	Apex to diaphragm every 10 mm
Window	-700/ 1000 HU
Field of View	(Target each lung 25 cm)

Normal HRCT
Septa absent
Vessel course short
Thinner the slice vessels become dots
Fissures identified as lines
Uniform gray lung parenchyma

Fig. 3.

CT for Chest Survey

Scan parameters	kVp 140, mas 180
Slice thickness	7 mm
Table feed	7-10 mm
Spiral length	30 sec
Recon interval	Based on the lesion
Recon algorithm	High-forlung, standard for mediastinum
Superior extent	Above lung apices
Inferior extent	Subdiaphragmatic –till adrenals
IV contrast	Hocm/locm 300 mg I/ml
Rate	3 ml/sec
Scan delay	20 seconds
Total volume	80-100 ml

Thoracic Evaluation for Hemoptysis

Scan parameters	kVp 140, mas 180
Slice thickness	5 mm
Table feed	5 mm/sec
Spiral length	30 sec
Recon interval	1-2 mm through pathology
Recon algorithm	High resolution
Superior extent	Lung apices
Inferior extent	Posterior costophrenic recess
IV contrast	None
Rate	-
Scan delay	-
Comments	Coronal MPRS, radial MPRS

Prone Scan (See Case 43)

This technique is sometimes needed to detect subtle density. This can be taken at the site of suspicion in the supine scan or routinely can be taken at 3 levels (aortic arch, carina, 3 cm above right hemidiaphragmatic) in case suspected clinically to have early restrictive lung disease with normal chest X-rays.

Expiratory Scan (See Case 46)

Expiratory CT techniques are used as adjunct to inspiratory scans in assessing patients with obstructive disease providing physiologic information in regards to regional lung function.

Post expiratory CT is useful in the diagnosis of disease charecterised by airflow limitation/airtrapping.

Focal, multifocal or diffuse airtrapping visible using these post-expiratory CT techniques are seen as areas of low attenuation and can confirm the presence of obstructive physiology in patients with airway abnormality visible on inspiratory scans.

Example: Emphysema, asthma, bronchiolitis.

NORMAL CT LUNG ANATOMY

An accurate understanding of normal lung anatomy along with pathological anatomical alterations in disease is essential in the interpretation of HRCT images (Refer to Tabular Column in page 10).

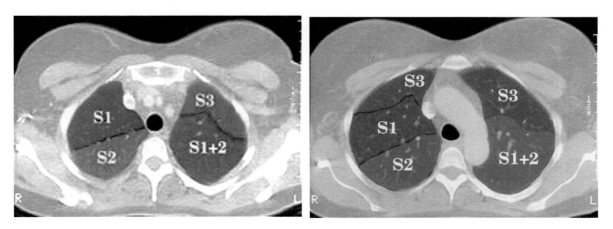

Fig. 4A   Fig. 4B

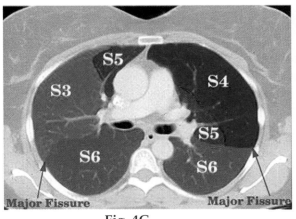

Fig. 4C

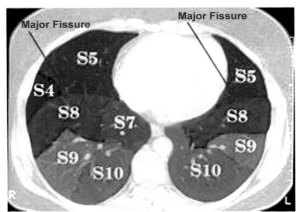

Fig. 4D

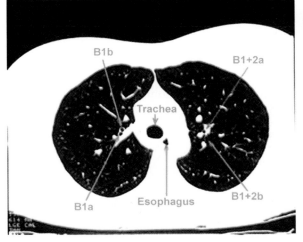

Fig. 4E

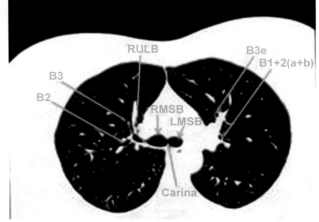

Fig. 4F

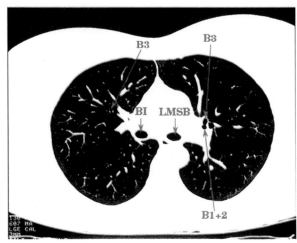

Fig. 4G

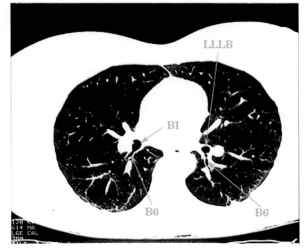

Fig. 4H

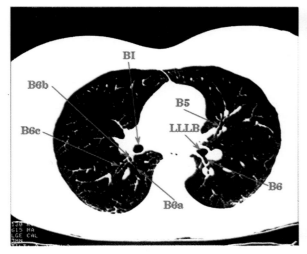

Fig. 4I

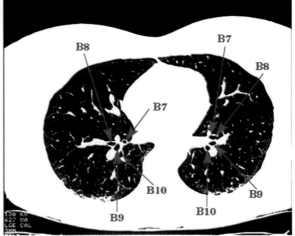

Fig. 4J

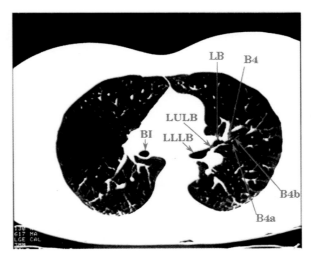

Fig. 4K

Right Lung

	Segment	Bronchus
Right Upper Lobe		
Apical	S1	B1
Posterior	S2	B2
Anterior	S3	B3
Right Middle Lobe		
Lateral	S4	B4
Medial	S5	B5
Right Lower Lobe		
Superior	S6	B6
Medial Basal	S7	B7
Anterior Basal	S8	B8
Lateral Basal	S9	B9
Posterior Basal	S10	B10
Left Lung		
Left Upper Lobe		
Apical Posterior	S1+2	B1+2
Anterior	S3	B3
Superior Lingular	S4	B4
Inferior Lingular	S5	B5
Left Lower Lobe		
Superior	S6	B6
Anterior Medial Basal	S8	B8
Lateral Basal	S9	B9
Posterior Basal	S10	B10

Anatomic Basis of Disease

The accurate interpretation of HRCT requires clear understanding of normal lung anatomy and pathological alterations in it.

The lung is maintained in a stable position within the chest by its hilar connection, to which the central or core structures are ultimately attached. The bronchovascular structures form the stem upon which the functional parenchyma are distributed.

LUNG PARENCHYMA

The parenchyma of the lung includes the pulmonary alveolar epithelium and capillary endothelium and the spaces between these structures, together with the tissues within the septa including the perivascular and perilymphatic tissues. More centrally it includes the peribronchiolar and peribronchial tissues.

The major core structures include pulmonary artery and its branches and the bronchi, which characteristically run in a parallel fashion. Both are enclosed within a connective tissue sheath, within which amorphous interstitial collagen, lymphatics and small lymph nodes can be found. The lung lymphatic system drains the visceral pleura and courses within the interlobular septa in parallel with septal veins.

There are approximately 23 generation of dichotomous branching in airways, from the trachea to the alveolar sac.

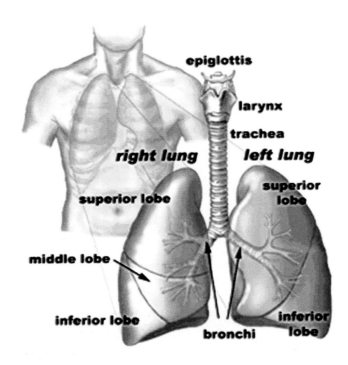

Fig. 5.

The division of the trachea gives rise to the left and right mainstem bronchi, which further divide into lobar and segmental bronchi. Segmental bronchi divide, and after 6 to 20 divisions they no longer contain cartilage in their walls and are referred to as bronchioles.

The trachea, bronchi and bronchioles down to the level of the terminal bronchiole constitute the purely conductive portion of the airway (Fig. 6).

The terminal bronchiole subdivide into respiratory bronchioles from which alveoli arise. Respiratory bronchioles give rise to alveolar ducts which give rise to alveolar sacs. These conduct air and also participate in gas exchange.

The central bronchi down to the segmental level can be identified routinely with 10-mm collimation CT sections, and 8th order branching airways can be seen with thin sections.

Airway diseases may be divided into those conditions affecting primarily the large airways, such as the trachea, main, lobar, and segmental bronchi, and those conditions primarily affecting smaller airways, particularly those airways less than 3 mm in size. Large airway diseases may be further subdivided into focal and diffuse airway abnormalities, primarily related to either narrowing or dilation.

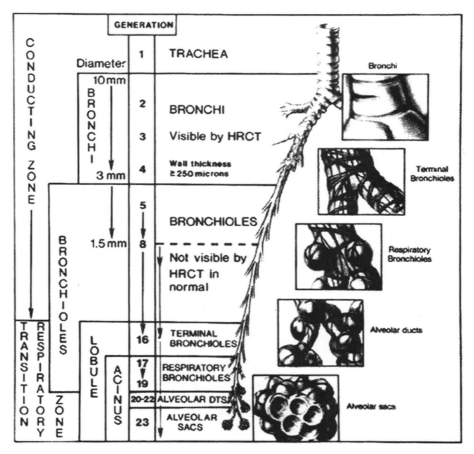

Fig. 6

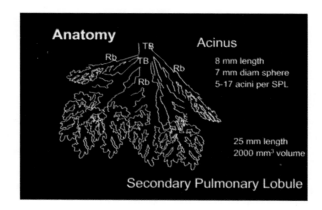

Fig. 7

Communication between adjacent alveoli occur through pores of Kohn, communication between distal bronchiole and alveoli occur through canals of Lambert.

Acinus – It is a unit of lung supplied by the terminal bronchiole, this typically include 3 respiratory bronchioles and their corresponding alveolar ducts and alveoli. An individual acinus measures 7-8 mm and is recognisable when filled with fluid or cells.

The most useful subsegmental unit of the lung in terms of HRCT is the secondary pulmonary lobule. It is a polyhedral structure that measures approximately 1-2.5 cm on each side, and is supplied by 3-5 terminal bronchioles, and therefore include 3-5 acini within the borders formed by interlobular septa. The secondary pulmonary lobule is divided into core and septal structures, the core structures include the pulmonary arteriole, terminal bronchiole, and accompanying lymphatics. The septal structures include pulmonary veins, lymphatics and the septum itself.

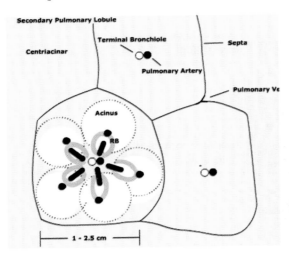
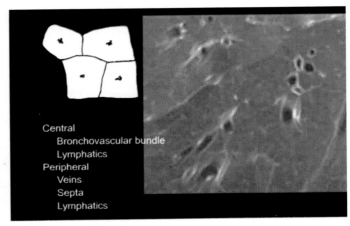

Fig. 8

Interlobular septae: Secondary lobules are marginated by septae which extend inward from the pleural surface. These septae are well defined in the anterior, lateral and diaphragmatic surface, they measure about 100 mmu (0.1 mm) in the subpleural location. Few normal septae are often visible on routine HRCT. They appear as thin straight lines of uniform thickness and are 1-2 cm long.

In central lung these septae are thinner and less well defined.

Lobular core: The HRCT appearances and the visibility of structures in the core are determined by the size. Secondary lobule is supplied by arteries and bronchioles that measure approximately 1 mm in diameter, intralobular bronchioles and arteries measure 0.7 mm. Acinar bronchioles and arteries measure 0.5 mm. The visible lobular core structures do not extend to the pleural surface.

Important rule to remember is that on routine HRCT intralobular bronchioles are not normally visible and bronchioles are normally not seen within 2-3 cm of pleural surface.

It is necessary to identify the peripheral pulmonary arteries to define the centre of the pulmonary lobule.

The substance of the secondary lobule which surrounds the lobular core and is contained within the interlobular septae consists of functioning lung parenchyma namely the alveoli, alveolar ducts, and vessels. This parenchyma is supported by a network of central and peripheral fibres to form a fibre skeleton of the lung.

INTERSTITIUM

Lung is supported by a network of connective tissue, called lung interstitium. This extends from the hila to the periphery of lung. This interstitium is not usually recognisable on HRCT and its clear visualisation depicts pathology. The interstitium is considered to have various components.

1. *Peribronchovascular interstitium* which is a system of fibers that invests the bronchi and pulmonary arteries. It extends from the hila to the periphery of the lung to invest the bronchioles and terminal arteries in the Secondary pulmonary lobules and is referred to as centrilobular interstitium.

THE LUNG INTERSTITIUM

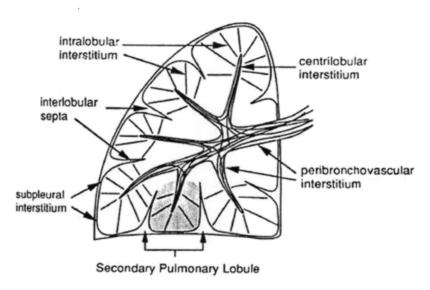

Fig. 9

2. *Subpleural interstitium* is located beneath the visceral pleura and envelops the lung in a fibrous sac. From this fibrous connective tissue, septae penetrate the lung parenchyma to form interlobular septa. These interlobular septa form the basic structure imaged in the periphery of the lung called the secondary pulmonary lobules.[12] The terms secondary pulmonary lobules, secondary lobule and pulmonary lobule are often used interchangeably. Secondary pulmonary lobules are irregular, polyhedral in shape and somewhat variable in size, measuring approximately 1-2.5 cm in diameter in most locations.

Secondary pulmonary lobule has got three main components:
- Interlobular septa,
- Centrilobular region,
- Lobular parenchyma and acinus.

a. Interlobular septa and contiguous subpleural interstitium: As mentioned above subpleural interstitium invests the lung with its extension into lung parenchyma to form interlobular septa, which contains terminal pulmonary veins and lymphatics. The veins are sometimes seen as linear or arcuate structures 5-10 mm from the centrilobular structures. The septa are better defined and visualised in the apical and anterior segment of the upper lobe, anterior and lateral aspects of middle lobe & lingula, diaphragmatic surface and along the mediastinal pleura. Within the central lung the interlobular septa are thinner and less well defined than the periphery.

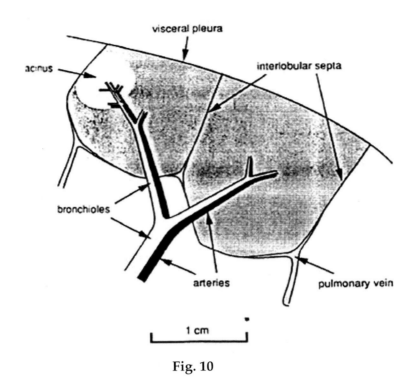

visceral pleura

acinus

interlobular septa

bronchioles

arteries

pulmonary vein

1 cm

Fig. 10

    b. Centrilobular region: The central portion of the secondary pulmonary lobule is referred to as centrilobular region or lobular core and contains the pulmonary artery and terminal bronchioles. It is invested with centrilobular interstitium, an extension of peribronchovascular interstitium. These usually appear as central linear, branching or dot like pattern in centre of secondary pulmonary lobule about one cm from the pleura.

    c. Lobular parenchyma and acinus: The substance of lung parenchyma within the pulmonary lobules consists of acini and intricate network of capillary beds. This vascular network along with walls of the acini and small airways are supported by a connective tissue stroma, a fine network of very thin fibers within the alveolar septa called the intralobular interstitium, or alveolar interstitium. This is invisible on HRCT in normal individuals. Pulmonary acini are the functioning structure of lung. There are a dozen or less of acini in each secondary pulmonary lobule, and vary in size measuring 6 to 10 mm each.

3. *Intralobular interstitium* that was referred by Weibel as septal fibers has been already described as a component of secondary pulmonary lobule.

Concept of Cortical and Medullary Lung

Cortical Lung

It consists of 3-4 rows of secondary pulmonary lobule forming a layer of 4 cm at the lung periphery and along the lung surface. Bronchi and pulmonary vessels are small at this level .

Medullary Lung

Pulmonary lobules in the central lung are smaller and more irregular in shape, parahilar vessels and bronchi are large and are easily seen on HRCT.

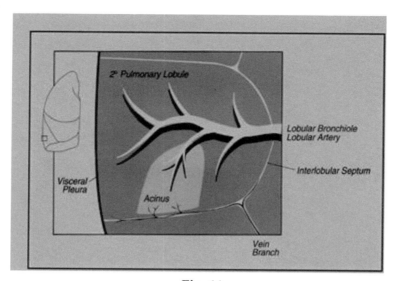

Fig. 11

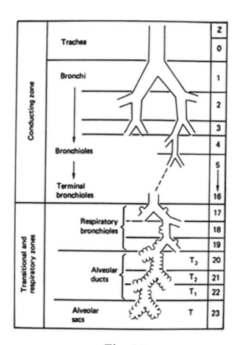

Fig. 12

Section 2

Overview of Lung Diseases

HRCT FINDINGS OF LUNG DISEASE

HRCT demonstrates various parenchymal diseases in a specific manner showing very high accuracy.

Generally HRCT findings of lung disease can be classified into four large categories based on their appearance. These include:

- Linear and reticular pattern opacities,
- Nodules and nodular opacities,
- Increased lung opacities and,
- Abnormalities associated with decreased lung opacity including cystic lesions, emphysema and airway abnormalities.

Linear and Reticular Opacities

Thickening of the interstitial network of the lung by fluid, fibrous tissue, or because of interstitial infiltration by cells or other material primarily results in an increase in linear or reticular lung opacities as seen on HRCT. Linear and reticular opacities can be manifested by the interface sign, peribronchovascular interstitial thickening, interlobular septal thickening, intralobular interstitial thickening, honeycombing, subpleural lines, centrilobular or lobular core abnormalities, and airway abnormalities.

Interface Sign

The presence of irregular interfaces between the aerated lung parenchyma and bronchi, vessels or the visceral pleural surface, has been termed interface sign by Zerhouni *et al*.

This sign is seen in patients with interstitial abnormalities regardless of cause. It is associated with increased lung reticulation. These linear opacities generally represent thickened inter and intralobular interstitial fibers. This sign is frequently seen in patients with fibrotic lung disease.

Peribronchovascular Interstitial Thickening

The thickened peribronchovascular interstitium cannot be distinguished from the underlying opacities of bronchial wall or pulmonary artery. This abnormality is perceived in HRCT as an increase in bronchial wall thickening (similar to peribronchial cuffing on chest X-ray) and an increase in the diameter of pulmonary artery branches.

Thickening of the parahilar peribronchovascular interstitium occurs in many diseases that cause a generalized interstitial abnormalities, which includes lymphangitic spread of carcinoma, interstitial pulmonary edema, and in diseases that lead on to pulmonary fibrosis such as sarcoidosis. It is also seen in 19% of patients with chronic hypersensitive pneumonitis.

Thickening of peribronchovascular interstitium can appear smooth, nodular, or irregular in different diseases. Smooth peribronchovascular interstitial thickening is most typical of patients with lymphangiitis carcinomatosa and interstitial pulmonary edema.

Nodular thickening of peribronchovascular interstitium is common in sarcoidosis and seen in lymphangitic carcinomatosa. Irregular peribronchovascular interstitial thickening is seen in patients with lung fibrosis. In case of extensive fibrosis, the interstitial thickening can appear as a conglomerate mass seen in patients with sarcoidosis, silicosis, or tuberculosis.

At times peribronchovascular interstitial thickening and fibrosis can lead to traction bronchiectasis. This can be differentiated from true bronchiectasis by pulmonary function test, absence of associated interstitial disease like nodules, honeycombing, etc and the absence of signet ring sign which is seen in true bronchiectasis as a result of bronchial wall thickening without thickening of the associated perivascular interstitium.

Interlobular Septal Thickening

This finding is commonly seen in patients with interstitial lung disease and easily recognized on HRCT. Septal thickening is seen in presence of interstitial fluids, cellular infiltrates, or fibrosis. The thickened interstitium is perpendicular to the pleura and outlines the structure of secondary pulmonary lobules and is usually 1-3 cm in length. When the thickened interlobular interstitium is involving multiple secondary lobules and seen in contact with the pleura, the term 'peripheral arcades', or 'polygonal arcades' are used.

Thickened interlobular septa also have been described using the terms 'septal lines', 'peripheral lines' and 'short lines'.

Septal thickening can be smooth, nodular, or irregular in contour in different pathological processes. Smooth interstitial thickening is seen in patients with pulmonary edema, lymphangitic spread of carcinoma, alveolar proteinosis, interstitial infiltrates with amyloidosis and few patients with pneumonia and in small percentage of patients with pulmonary fibrosis. Nodular or beaded septal thickening occurs in patients with lymphangiitis carcinomatosa or lymphoma, sarcoidosis, silicosis, coal workers pneumoconiosis and amyloidosis.

Parenchymal Band

The term parenchymal band has been used to describe non-tapering, reticular opacities, from 2-5 cm in length that can be seen in patients with pulmonary fibrosis or other causes of interstitial thickening. These lines are usually peripheral and contact the pleura. Parenchymal bands are more commonly a result of contiguous septal lines or occasionally a result of peribronchovascular fibrosis, coarse scars or atelectasis associated with lung or pleural fibrosis.

Parenchymal bands have been reported most commonly in patients with asbestos related lung (upto 60%) in association with pleural thickening, sarcoidosis with interstitial fibrosis, silicosis associated with progressive massive fibrosis and conglomerate masses, and tuberculosis.

Subpleural Interstitial Thickening

Thickening of subpleural interstitium is a finding usually seen along with the diseases, which causes septal thickening. Identification of subpleural thickening is usually difficult as the interstitium is usually adjacent to the pleura and chest wall, however along the fissures this abnormality appears more prominent due to the double subpleural layer and the adjacent lung interface.

In general the differentials for subpleural interstitial thickening is the same as interlobular septal thickening however it is more commonly seen in patients with idiopathic pulmonary fibrosis and usual pulmonary fibrosis of any cause. It is also seen in collagen vascular disease and drug reaction.

Nodular thickening of subpleural interstitium is seen in patients with lymphangiitis carcinomatosa, sarcoidosis and silicosis.

Intralobular Interstitial Thickening

Thickening of the intralobular interstitium results in a fine reticular pattern as seen on HRCT with the lines of opacity separated by a few mm. This finding may or may not be present with interlobular or subpleural interstitial thickening. However very small honeycomb cysts or dilated bronchioles with adjacent pulmonary fibrosis is a common association.

Intralobular interstitial thickening or small reticular pattern are commonly seen with idiopathic pulmonary fibrosis and other causes of usual interstitial pneumonia (UIP) such as rheumatoid arthritis, scleroderma, and other collagen vascular diseases and it appears to predominantly involve the peripheral acini resulting in 'peripheral acinar distribution'. Other causes of intralobular interstitial thickening include asbestosis, chronic hypersensitivity pneumonitis and alveolar proteinosis.

Honeycombing

Extensive interstitial and alveolar fibrosis that results in alveolar disruption and bronchiectasis produces the classic and characteristic appearance of honeycombing or honeycomb lung.

Pathologically honeycombing is defined by the presence of small air containing cystic spaces of about 1 cm in diameter, and generally lined by bronchial epithelium and having thickened wall composed of dense fibrous tissue measuring 1-3 mm. Honeycombing indicates the End stage lung disease.

Honeycombing predominates in the peripheral and subpleural lung region and spares the parahilar parenchyma.

Honeycombing is seen in patients with Usual interstitial pneumonia associated with IPF or rheumatoid lung, asbestosis, sarcoidosis and hypersensitive pneumonitis. Honeycombing is associated with other features of lung fibrosis.

Subpleural Lines

A curvilinear opacity a few mm thick, less than 1 cm from the pleural surface, and paralleling the pleura is described as subpleural lines.

Subpleural lines are a result of confluence of peribronchiolar interstitial abnormalities in patients with asbestosis, which represent early fibrosis with associated alveolar flattening and collapse. Subpleural lines are seen primarily in asbestosis, scleroderma and at times in normal patients which are the result of dependent density.

Centrilobular Abnormalities

Centrilobular linear or reticular abnormalities can reflect interstitial thickening or bronchiolar abnormalities such as bronchiolar dilatation and the finding of 'tree-in-bud'.

a. Interstitial thickening: Diseases that cause interstitial thickening often result in prominence of centrilobular vessels, which appears as a dot, Y-shaped, or X-shaped branching opacity. This finding represents the thickening of centrilobular interstitium and is seen in patients with lymphangitic spread of carcinoma and lymphoma, interstitial pulmonary edema and lung fibrosis.
b. Bronchiolar dilatation and tree-in-bud appearance: The intralobular bronchiole, which is not seen in normal subjects is sometimes visible on HRCT in patients with centrilobular interstitial thickening because of a combination of increased attenuation of surrounding lung, thickening of peribronchiolar interstitium and dilatation of bronchioles which occurs as a result of fibrosis.

In some patients small airways that are dilated and/or filled with pus, mucus or inflammatory exudate appear as small, well-defined, centrilobular nodular, linear, or branching structures of soft tissue opacity referred to as tree-in-bud or budding tree appearance. These findings are seen in patients with Asian panbronchiolitis, endobronchial spread of tuberculosis, cystic fibrosis, bronchopneumonia, bronchiectasis of any cause and other airway diseases that result in accumulation of mucus and pus within small bronchi.

Nodules and Nodular Opacities

The diagnosis of nodular opacities are based on their size and distribution:

Small Nodules

These include round opacities of less than one centimeter in diameter. Many authors have described nodules less than three millimeters as micronodules, however this classification has not proved to be of any value in differentiation of disease pathology. Small nodules can arise from two basic structures, either predominantly from the interstitium or from the air space.

Nodules considered to be interstitial are usually well-defined and are of soft tissue attenuation obscuring the edges of the vessels or other structures they touch. Interstitial nodules are commonly seen in sarcoidosis, histiocytosis X, silicosis, miliary TB, metastasis and coal workers' pneumoconiosis.

Air space nodules are usually ill-defined and can be of soft tissue density or less dense (ground glass opacities). Air space nodules have also been termed as acinar nodules because they approximate the size of acini but they are not truly acinar. Small nodules can be randomly distributed, perilymphatic in distribution or predominantly centrilobular.

i. Random distribution: Small nodules that appear randomly distributed in relation to structures of the secondary lobule are often seen in patients with miliary TB and miliary fungal infections. Hematogenous spread of metastasis is randomly distributed however, may show preponderance for lung periphery and bases[31] and at times, a relationship with vessels is observed. Histiocytosis X and silicosis may show random distribution when numerous. However they usually present with specific locations.

ii. Perilymphatic distribution: Nodules that predominate in relation to the parahilar peribronchovascular interstitium, the centrilobular interstitium, interlobular septa and in a subpleural location are typical of patients with sarcoidosis, silicosis and coal worker's pneumoconiosis, and lymphangitic spread of carcinoma. Each of these diseases typically results in histological abnormalities that occur in relation to lymphatics.

In sarcoidosis, HRCT shows nodules of 1 mm to 1 cm or more. Nodules are usually peribronchovascular or subpleural in location but less commonly septal or centrilobular. At times lung nodules of 1-4 cm are seen which represent masses of granulomatous tissue. Sarcoid nodules show upper lobe predominance and the large nodules may cavitate.

In silicosis and coal workers' pneumoconiosis the nodules are of 2-5 mm in diameter which predominate at centrilobular and subpleural locations. Less frequently nodules are seen in relation to peribronchovascular interstitium and interlobular septa. These nodules are diffusely distributed but have upper lobe predominance. Calcification of nodules are not uncommon.

In patients with lymphangitic spread of carcinoma, nodules are visible most often in the thickened peribronchovascular interstitium and interlobular septae. Septal thickening with nodularity may give an appearance of 'beaded septum'. Subpleural nodules are not as profuse as in sarcoid.

iii. Centrilobular distribution: These nodules may be dense and homogenous or of ground glass opacity. They are usually associated with other interstitial signs however, may occur solitarily. The nodules are few mm to a cm in size and seen in the center of secondary pulmonary lobules, and are evenly spread. Centrilobular nodules reflect the presence of either interstitial or air space abnormalities. Well-defined small peribronchial nodules are seen in patients with histiocytosis X. Ill-defined centrilobular opacities can occur in patients with endobronchial spread of tuberculosis or non-tubercular mycobacterium (usually tree-in-bud appearance is seen), Asian panbronchiolitis, hypersensitivity pneumonitis (ground glass appearance seen), asbestosis and bronchoalveolar carcinoma.

Large Nodules

These include nodules of more than 1 cm in diameter. The term mass is used for nodules of more than 3 cm in diameter. Many conditions that cause small nodules may progress to develop large nodules. Nodules may coalesce with each other forming conglomerate masses or nodules.

In 50% of patients with sarcoidosis confluent nodules are seen. These are usually peribronchovascular, irregular and associated with traction bronchiectasis. 29% of patients with histiocytosis X show large nodules.

In progressive fibrotic lung disease large masses of fibrous tissue surround the bronchi within the central and perihilar lung. The bronchi may show collapse as a result of mass effect or dilatation due to traction bronchiectasis. Similar findings can be seen in post treatment tuberculosis.

Patients with silicosis and coal workers' pneumoconiosis which have developed progressive massive fibrosis show evidence of conglomerate mass typically in the upper lobe with absence of traction bronchiectasis, however areas of emphysema adjacent to the conglomerate mass is common.

Focal fibrotic masses as a result of asbestos exposure are considered to be a result of round atelectasis or fibrotic scarring. Round atelectasis occurs most commonly in posterior lung or paravertebral region. It is associated with folding of lung and volume loss with traction of bronchi and vessels towards it giving an appearance of 'comet tail'. Round atelectasis may show an air bronchogram.

Increased Lung Opacities

Increased lung opacity or parenchymal opacification is a common finding on HRCT in patients with chronic lung disease. Increased lung opacities are generally described as ground glass opacity, consolidation and calcification.

Ground Glass Opacities

This finding on HRCT appears as a hazy increase in lung opacity that is not associated with obstruction of the underlying vessel. Ground glass opacity reflects minimal thickening of the septal or alveolar interstitium, thickening of alveolar walls, or the presence of cells or fluid partially filling the alveolar spaces. Ground glass opacities can be geographic involving only a certain segment of the lung, or it can involve the entire lobule or at times it may involve the centrilobular region, giving the appearance of ill-defined centrilobular nodules. The presence of air-filled bronchus that appear too black within an area of lung can also be a clue as to the presence of ground glass opacities. Ground glass opacity is highly a significant finding and it often indicates the presence of an ongoing, active and potentially a treatable process. At times ground glass opacity may suggest the presence of fibrosis.

The most common causes include usual interstitial pneumonia, bronchiolitis obliterans organizing pneumonia, sarcoidosis and hypersensitivity pneumonitis. Other causes include pneumonia, alveolar proteinosis, acute interstitial pneumonia and other causes of diffuse alveolar damage.

Consolidation

Increased lung attenuation with obstruction of underlying pulmonary vessel is referred to as consolidation. Air bronchograms may be present.

Consolidation is seen in disease that replace the alveolar air by fluid, cells, tissue or other material but diseases that produce extensive, confluent interstitial abnormalities such as usual interstitial pneumonia and sarcoidosis can also produce consolidation pattern. The differential diagnosis of consolidation include pneumonia of different causes, bronchiolitis obliterans organizing pneumonia, hypersensitivity pneumonitis, eosinophilic pneumonia, radiation pneumonia, bronchoalveolar carcinoma and lymphoma, alveolar proteinosis, acute interstitial pneumonia, sarcoidosis, drug reaction and ARDS.

Lung Calcification and Increased Lung Opacity

Multifocal lung calcification, often associated with lung nodules has been reported in association with infectious granulomatous disease such as tuberculosis, sarcoidosis, silicosis, talcosis, amyloidosis, and fat embolism associated with ARDS.

Diffuse and dense lung calcification can be seen in presence of metastatic calcification, disseminated pulmonary ossification, or alveolar microlithiasis. Diffuse and increased lung attenuation in the absence of calcification can be seen as a result of amiodarone lung toxicity.

An entity called metastatic calcification is referred to deposition of calcium within lung parenchyma which can occur due to hypercalcemia in patients with abnormal calcium and phosphate metabolism and is most common in patients with chronic renal failure and secondary hyperparathyroidism. Metastatic calcification is typically interstitial and can be associated with secondary lung fibrosis.

Alveolar microlithiasis is a term used for widespread intra-alveolar calcification so called microlith or calcosphere. These microliths have a posterior and lower lobe preponderance with a high concentration in subpleural, parenchymal, intralobular and centrilobular interstitium.

Decreased Lung Opacities and Cystic Abnormalities

A variety of abnormalities result in decreased lung attenuation or air-filled cystic lesions in HRCT. These include honeycombing, bronchiectasis, emphysema, lung cysts, cavitary nodules, mosaic perfusion, and air trapping due to airway diseases.

Honeycombing

This finding is described before under linear and reticular opacities.

At times large subpleural cystic spaces, several centimeters in diameter, can be associated with honeycombing, mimicking the appearance of bullae.

Lung Cysts

These are thin walled (less than 3 mm), well-defined and circumscribed, air containing lesion. These cysts are lined by one of the variety of cellular elements, usually fibrous or epithelial in nature.

Lung cysts are typically seen in Lymphangiomyomatosis (LAM) and Histiocytosis X. In patients with histiocytosis X the cysts have a bizarre shapes and are usually thicker walled than the cysts in LAM which are rounder and more uniform in distribution.

Lung cysts should be differentiated from emphysematous bullae, blebs and pneumatocele.

Emphysema

Emphysema is defined as a permanent, abnormal enlargement of air spaces distal to the terminal bronchiole, accompanied by the destruction of the walls of the involved air spaces. In HRCT emphysema appears as focal areas of very low attenuation that can easily be contrasted with the surrounding, higher attenuation normal lung parenchyma.

Emphysema can be classified into centrilobular, panlobular, paraseptal and cicatricial emphysema based on its HRCT finding.

Centrilobular (proximal or centriacinar) emphysema is characterised by presence of multiple small lucencies which predominate in the upper lobes. This pattern lacks a visible wall and if walls are occasionally seen they relate to areas of fibrosis.

Panlobular (panacinar) emphysema typically results in an overall decrease in lung attenuation, and a reduction in size of the pulmonary vessels, without the focal areas of lucency. Areas of panlobular emphysema typically lack visible walls.

Paraseptal (distal or peripheral) emphysema result in the presence of subpleural lucencies which often share a very thin walls that are barely visible on HRCT.

Cicatrical (irregular air space enlargements) emphysema can be seen in patients with fibrosis.

-24-

Bullae and Blebs

Bullae has been defined as a sharply demarcated area of emphysema measuring more than 1 cm (upto 20 cm) and having a distinct thin wall of less than 1 mm in thickness. They are usually associated with emphysema. When emphysema is associated with predominant bullae, it may be termed bullous emphysema.

The term bleb is used to describe a gas containing space within the visceral pleura.

Pneumatocele

Pneumatocele is defined as a thin-walled, gas-filled space within the lung, usually occurring in association with acute pneumonia and almost invariably transient. Based on HRCT alone pneumatocele cannot be differentiated from lung cyst or bullae, but the clinical finding of lung infection suggests the possibility of the former.

Cavitatory Nodules

Cavitatory nodules have a thicker and more irregular walls than do lung cysts. They are seen in histiocytosis X, tuberculosis, fungal infection, sarcoidosis, rheumatoid lung, septic embolism, metastatic tumor, Wegener's granulomatosis, etc.

Bronchiectasis

Bronchiectasis is generally defined as localized, irreversible bronchial dilatation. It usually occurs due to chronic infection, but airway obstruction by tumor, impacted material, or inherited abnormalities can also play a significant role.

Cylindrical bronchiectasis the mildest form of this disease is characterized by presence of thick-walled bronchi, which extend into the lung periphery and fail to show normal tapering. Depending on the orientation of the scanned bronchi, it may show tram track or signet ring sign.

Varicose bronchiectasis shows a similar pattern to cylindrical bronchiectasis but the bronchial walls are more irregular and assume a beaded appearance, termed string of pearls.

Cystic bronchiectasis most often appears as a group or cluster of air fluid cysts, but cysts can also be fluid filled giving the appearance of cluster of grapes.

Knowing the various presentation patterns of parenchymal lesions in HRCT, we can diagnose specific diseases using this modality.

CLASSIFICATION BASED ON ETIOLOGY

Interstitial lung diseases can be classified based on the specific causative pathology into,
1. Infective causes

Viral	Bacterial	Protozoa	Fungal
CMV	Miliary TB	PCP (IC)	Histoplasmosis
Herpes simplex	Brucellosis	Toxoplasma gondii (IC)	Coccidiodes
Varicella Zoster	Other mycobacterial		Cryptococcus
Infectious mononucleosis			Aspergillosis

2. Inflammatory
   - Sarcoidosis
   - Histiocytosis X
   - Eosinophilic granuloma
3. Collagen vascular disease
   - Rheumatoid lung
   - SLE
   - Scleroderma
   - Ankylosing spondylitis
   - Sjogren's syndrome
   - Dermatomyositis
4. Inhalation of particulate matter
   Organic

From Fungi	Farmer's lung	Mouldy Hay
	Bagassosis	Mouldy Bagasse
	Mushroom worker's lung	Mushroom compost
From avian protein	Pigeon fancier lung	Dropping
	Budgerigar	Droppings
From mammalian protein	Pituitary snuff taker's lung	
	Rat handler's lung	Rat urine/serum

   Inorganic
   - Silicosis
   - Asbestosis
   - Coal worker's pneumoconiosis
   - Others, e.g. stannosis, siderosis
5. Fibrosing allergic alveolitis
   - Cytogenic
   - Secondary
6. Drugs/poisons/toxic fumes
   - Cytotoxic drugs (e.g. Bleomycin, Busulfan, Vincristine, Methotrexate, Adriamycin and Cremastin)
   - Non-cytotoxic drugs (e.g. Nitrofurantoin, Amiodarone, Gold and Penicillamine)
7. Alveolar proteinosis and pulmonary alveolar microlithiasis
8. Malignancy
   - Lymphangitic carcinomatosa
   - Kaposis sarcoma (Immunocompromised)
   - Lymphoma → NHL (Immunocompromised)
   - Hematogenous metastasis
9. Benign
   - Neurofibromatosis
   - Lymphangiomyomatosis
   - Tuberous sclerosis

10. Systemic Vasculitides
- PAN
- Wegener's granulomatosis
- Systemic necrotizing vasculitides

11. Pulmonary Eosinophilia
- As a response to infections → parasitic, fungi
- Loeffler's syndrome
- Filariasis
- Allergic bronchopulmonary aspergillosis

12. Miscellaneous
- Lymphocytic interstitial pneumonitis
- Nonspecific interstitial pneumonitis
- Pulmonary edema
- Amyloidosis
- Idiopathic pulmonary hemosiderosis

ANATOMIC PATTERNS AND PATHOLOGICAL CORRELATES IN PARENCHYMATOUS LUNG DISEASE

Normal Pattern

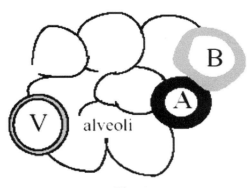

Fig. 1

Intra-alveolar Pattern

This is the classic pattern of bacterial lobar and lobular pneumonias. It is also seen in aspiration pneumonia and in uncommon conditions such as pulmonary alveolar proteinosis, Goodpasture's syndrome, and idiopathic pulmonary hemosiderosis. In this pattern, the alveolar spaces are occupied by materials that give the water-density opacities referred to as "infiltrates".

Condition	Cause of infiltrate
Goodpasture's syndrome	Blood
Bacterial pneumonias	Neutrophils
Pulmonary edema and Pneumocystis pneumonia	Thin serous fluid
Pulmonary alveolar proteinosis	Viscous gelatinous substance
Loeffler's syndrome	Eosinophils
Hemosiderosis	Macrophages
Organizing bacterial and aspiration pneumonias	Fibrous connective tissue

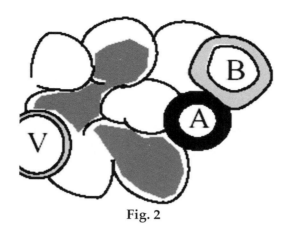

Fig. 2

Clinical Correlate

In terms of pulmonary functional effects, intra-alveolar lesions tend to affect pulmonary venous blood oxygen tension due to shunting produced by abnormal ventilation/perfusion balance.

Because CO_2 is more readily diffusable through water than O_2, one would expect hypoxemia to dominate the results of clinical arterial blood gas measurements. Hypercapnia should then be considered a dire message that the disease process is *in extremis.*

Some potentially fatal intra-alveolar diseases, notably acute bacterial pneumonia, produce death more through the systemic toxic effects of microbial and inflammatory byproducts than through specific embarrassment of pulmonary function.

Interstitial Pattern

In this pattern, substances remain confined to the interstitium, not involving the alveoli. Interstitium is intrinsically much less voluminous than the alveolar spaces - much less fluid, exudate, or other abnormal materials may accumulate there to produce an equivalent pathophysiologic effect on gas exchange. Therefore, the radiographic expression for a given level of functional embarrassment may be less severe for interstitial than for intra-alveolar lesions.

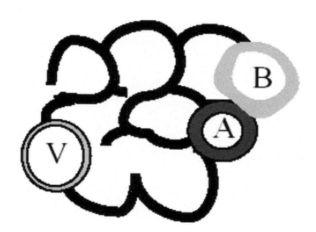

Fig. 3

Abnormal substances found in the interstitium

Substance	Condition
Serous fluid	Diffuse alveolar damage [DAD]-ARDS
Lymphocytes	Viral pneumonias, usual interstitial pneumonia, lymphocytic interstitial pneumonia
Plasma cells	Collagen vascular diseases
Macrophages	Sarcoidosis
Fibrous connective tissue	Interstitial fibrosis, "honeycomb lung"

Clinical Correlate

When an interstitial process involves only fluid and inflammatory cells, shunting of unoxygenated blood through the abnormal areas results in hypoxemia without significant hypercapnia.

When, however, the interstitium becomes fibrotic through ingrowth of fibroblasts and collagen, the lung becomes less deformable and may not expand normally in inspiration. In such a case, the result is a *ventilatory* deficit due to a *restrictive* (rather than obstructive) mechanism. Here, hypercapnia accompany hypoxemia.

Combination Intra-alveolar/interstitial Pattern

There are some conditions which tend to demonstrate a mixture of the intra-alveolar and interstitial patterns. The most important of these is **diffuse alveolar damage** (DAD), the anatomic correlate of clinical **adult respiratory distress syndrome** (ARDS).

Less common conditions with a similar pattern are **desquamative interstitial pneumonia** (DIP), in which macrophages fill the alveoli, and **eosinophilic pneumonia**, in which eosinophils predominate.

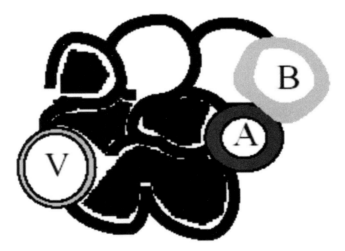

Fig. 4

Cinical Correlate

Most of these conditions present acutely and result in rapid hypoxemia.

1. Diagnostic data sheet for diffuse lung disease

NAME: AGE/SEX: HOSPITAL NO.

ADDRESS:

DIAGNOSIS:

FOLLOW-UP:

Chest X-ray	Upper zone	Middle zone	Lower zone	Peripheral	Central
Reticular lines					
Reticulonodular					
Nodular					
Confluencing shadows					
Septal lines					
Ground glass opacity					
Air bronchogram					
Honeycombing					
Increased lucency					
Pleural effusion					
Lymph nodes					
Hilar mass					
ETC					

FOCAL LUNG DISEASES (Fig. 5)

Introduction

Focal pulmonary lesions are among the most common findings in everyday radiology practice. At imaging, focal lung disease may present as nodular opacity or localized area of consolidation.

Causes of focal lung disease include malignant lesions such as bronchogenic carcinoma, solitary metastases and carcinoid tumors; benign tumors such as granuloma, hamartoma; vascular processes; and focal areas of inflammation.

Modern imaging techniques are of paramount importance in the detection and the classification of focal abnormalities of the lung parenchyma. Compared to plain chest films, CT offers the advantage of providing unique morphologic clues that may help characterize focal pulmonary processes.

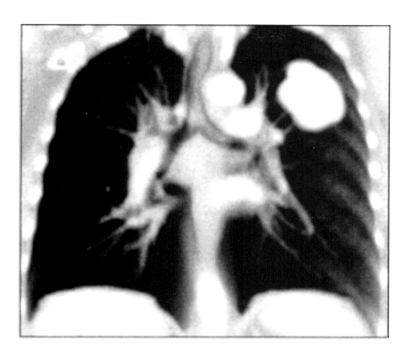

Fig. 5: Focal lung lesion

IMAGING FEATURES THAT AID IN THE IDENTIFICATION OF BENIGN AND MALIGNANT FOCAL ABNORMALITY

Lesion Size

Lesions with diameters of more than 3 cm are more likely malignant whereas those with diameters less than 3 cm may be assumed to be benign.

Lesion Growth

It has been shown that malignant tumors have tumor-doubling time between 30 and 490 days. Tumor doubling, in this context, refers to doubling of the volume and not doubling of the diameter. Therefore, the spherical lesion with a diameter of 1 cm that doubles its volume reaches a diameter, after the doubling, of 1.25 cm.

Assuming a tumor doubling time of 360 days for a malignant lesion, it becomes clear that the tumor growth may be extremely difficult to detect using plain film radiography.

Margins

The margins of solitary pulmonary lesions are categorized into four types, smooth, moderately smooth, slightly irregular, and grossly irregular with spiculations.

Lesion Texture

The presence and nature of calcification is undoubtedly one of the most important features that help distinguish benign from malignant disease. Nevertheless, only specific patterns of calcifications are associated with benign disease. These patterns include the central nidus, the laminated pattern, the popcorn-like pattern, and diffuse calcification. In contrast, eccentric or fine-stippled calcification as well as amorphous calcifications cannot be regarded as reliable indicators of benign disease since they are also seen in malignant disorders.

Cavitation

Lesions in which the thickest part of the cavity wall was 1 mm thick are considered benign; lesions where the cavity wall is over 15 mm in thickness, malignant.

Contrast Enhancement

Malignant lesions usually have an enhancement of greater than 20 HU after injection of contrast material.

Biological Activity

FDG-PET imaging may demonstrate focal hypermetabolism as a parameter of malignancy and exclude malignant disease when such focal hypermetabolism is not present. With the new generation of PET scanners, the sensitivity of PET imaging appears to be good enough to reliably depict lesions as small as 1 cm.

Differential diagnosis of SPN
Malignant tumors
Bronchogenic, metastatic, carcinoid
Hamartomas
Granulomas
TB, histoplasmosis, coccidioidomycosis, cryptococcosis
Other
AVM's, Dirofilaria immitis, RA nodule, infarct, hematoma, sarcoidosis, rounded atlectasis, pseudotumor

Halosign

Halosign by definition is a discrete nodule surrounded by a circular margin of ground glass attenuation representing edema or hemorrhage. Seen in invasive pulmonary aspergillosis, leukemia, CMV, Kaposis.

Positive Bronchus Sign

Presence of air bronchogram is an important finding in solitary nodules, many studies have shown pulmonary lesions that directly abut, displace, or narrow a bisible bronchial lumen were invariably malignant.

Feeding Vessel Sign

Focal diseases in which identification of feeding vessels adjacent to nodules have been described in metastasis, infarcts, AVM.

FOCAL LUNG DISEASES

Cavities

Neoplastic	Primary lung carcinoma, Hodgkins lymphoma, squamous metastasis.
Infective	Abscess, septic emboli, fungal diseases,TB, pneumatocele
Noninfective granulomatous	Wegener's, rheumatoid, PMF, sarcoid
Vascular	Infarct, hematoma, traumatic lung cyst
Congenital	Sequestration, bronchogenic cyst
Mimickers	Bowel herniation, bulla, cystic bronchiectasis, honeycombing

Solitary Masses and Nodules

Neoplastic	Primary lung carcinoma, melaris-sarcoma, RCC, seminoma, benign hamartoma, adenoma
Infective	Organizing pneumonia, tuberculoma, fungal, hydatid
Noninfective granulomatous	Caplans, Wegener's, rheumatoid
Vascular	AVM, hematoma, infarct
Congenital	Sequestration, bronchogenic cyst
Mimickers	Skin lesions, artifacts, loculated effusion, mediastinal masses

DIFFUSE LUNG DISEASES

Many different disease processes may present with diffuse lung shadowing on chest radiography. These processes include infection, neoplasm, pulmonary edema, hemorrhage, environmental and occupational lung diseases, drug-induced lung disease, aspiration pneumonia, many forms of interstitial lung diseases (ILDs). "Diffuse" implies involvement of all lobes of both lungs, but the process need not affect all lobes or all lung regions uniformly. Although most disorders with diffuse lung shadowing will be parenchymal processes, some airway diseases such as bronchiectasis and cystic fibrosis may present with diffuse lung infiltrates. Similarly, some vascular disorders such as pulmonary veno-occlusive disease are associated with diffuse lung infiltrates and may be mistaken for ILD.

A clinician trying to determine the best diagnostic approach to a patient with diffuse lung infiltrates detected on chest radiography or HRCT should focus on 3 pivotal parameters to narrow the differential diagnosis and guide the diagnostic evaluation.

Pivotal Parameters in the Diagnosis of Diffuse Lung Disease

- Tempo of disease
- Radiological pattern
- Distribution
- Associated radiological findings
- Clinical context

TEMPO OF DISEASE

Acute (less than 4 to 6 weeks in duration)

Diffuse lung diseases with an acute onset most commonly include:-

    Infection (pneumonia)

    Pulmonary edema (cardiogenic or noncardiogenic)

    Pulmonary hemorrhage, or aspiration.

Some diffuse infiltrative lung diseases or ILDs may also present acutely

    Hypersensitivity pneumonitis

    Drug-induced lung disease

    Pneumonitis related to toxic exposures

    Acute eosinophilic pneumonia

    Acute interstitial pneumonia

    Cryptogenic organizing pneumonia

    Idiopathic bronchiolitis obliterans with organizing pneumonia.

Chronic

Most chronic diffuse lung diseases are ILDs which show a slow tempo of progression over many months or even years.

- IPF
- Sarcoidosis
- Connective tissue disorders
- Pneumoconioses
- Hypersensitivity pneumonitis
- Drug-induced diseases.

RADIOLOGICAL PATTERN

HRCT contributes to the differential diagnosis of diffuse lung disease on the basis of the recognition of the main pattern, associated findings and distribution of the lesions.

    Six main categories of features may be described at CT:

- Reticular pattern
- Nodular patterns
- Bronchocentric pattern
- Angiocentric pattern
- Increased lung attenuation
- Decreased lung attenuation.

    The distribution of the lesions is assessed not only at the regional level including vertical (upper, middle, lower) and axial (cortical/medullar, anterior/posterior) distribution, but also at the level of the secondary pulmonary lobule. Associated lesions include abnormality of the airways and pulmonary vessels, pleural thickening, effusion or calcification, hilar and mediastinal lymphadenopathy.

Classification of Diffuse Lung Diseases according to Radiological Pattern

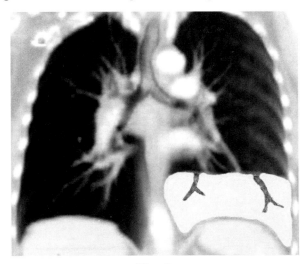

Fig. 6

Consolidation

Acute: Infection, acute respiratory distress syndrome, hemorrhage, aspiration, acute eosinophilic pneumonia, acute interstitial pneumonia, cryptogenic organizing pneumonia (also called idiopathic bronchiolitis obliterans with organizing pneumonia [BOOP])

Chronic: Chronic infections (tuberculosis, fungal), chronic eosinophilic pneumonia, cryptogenic organizing pneumonia, lymphoproliferative diseases, bronchioloalveolar carcinoma, pulmonary alveolar proteinosis.

Linear or Reticular Opacities

Acute: Infections (viral, mycoplasma), pulmonary edema.

Chronic: Idiopathic pulmonary fibrosis (IPF) or usual interstitial pneumonia, connective tissue disease–associated pulmonary fibrosis, asbestosis, sarcoidosis, hypersensitivity pneumonitis, drug-induced lung disease.

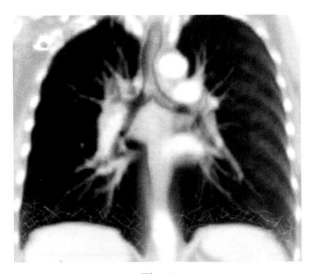

Fig. 7

Small Nodules (Round Opacities < 1 cm in diameter)

Acute: Infections (disseminated tuberculosis, fungal or viral infections), hypersensitivity pneumonitis (poorly circumscribed, centrilobular).

Chronic: Sarcoidosis, hypersensitivity pneumonitis, silicosis, coal worker's pneumoconiosis, respiratory bronchiolitis, metastases, alveolar microlithiasis.

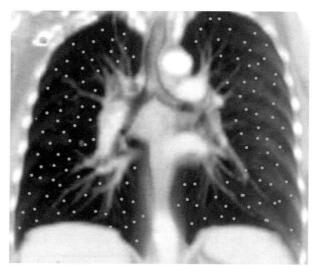

Fig. 8

Cystic Air Spaces

Acute: Pneumocystis carinii pneumonia, septic embolism.

Chronic: Pulmonary Langerhans cell histiocytosis, pulmonary lymphangioleiomyomatosis, honeycomb lung caused by IPF or other disorders, metastatic disease (rare).

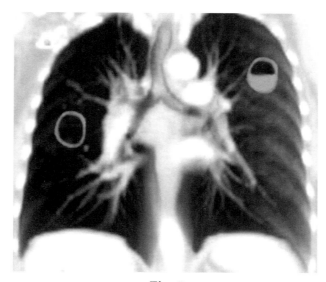

Fig. 9

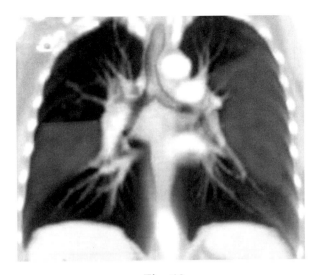

Fig. 10

Ground Glass Opacities

Acute: Infections (*P carinii*, cytomegalovirus), pulmonary edema, hemorrhage, hypersensitivity pneumonitis, acute inhalational exposures, drug-induced lung diseases, acute interstitial pneumonia.

Chronic: Nonspecific interstitial pneumonia (idiopathic or related to underlying diseases, e.g. connective tissue diseases), respiratory bronchiolitis–associated interstitial lung disease, desquamative interstitial pneumonia, drug-induced lung diseases, pulmonary alveolar proteinosis.

Thickened Interlobular Septa

Acute: Pulmonary edema.

Chronic: Lymphangitic carcinomatosis, pulmonary alveolar proteinosis, sarcoidosis, pulmonary veno-occlusive disease.

Bronchocentric
Suggestive of sarcoidosis, lymphangitic carcinomatosis, lymphoma or Kaposi's sarcoma.

Angiocentric
- Primary and secondary vasculitis
- Angioinvasive infection
- IV drug abuse
- Metastatic cancer

Chronic Lung Scarring

Findings which indicate fibrosis and lung destruction, in addition to thickening of the interstitium, include:
1. Architectural distortion
2. Honeycombing
3. Cicatricial bronchiectasis
4. Thin-walled cystic spaces.

Distribution

Upper lung predominance: Pulmonary Langerhans' cell histiocytosis, silicosis, coal worker's pneumoconiosis, carmustine-related pulmonary fibrosis, reactivation tuberculosis, *P. carinii* pneumonia on pentamidine prophylaxis.

Lower lung predominance: IPF, pulmonary fibrosis associated with connective tissue diseases, asbestosis, chronic aspiration.

Central (perihilar) predominance: Sarcoidosis, berylliosis.

Peripheral predominance: IPF, chronic eosinophilic pneumonia, cryptogenic organizing pneumonia (or idiopathic BOOP).

Associated Radiological Findings

Pleural effusion or thickening: Pulmonary edema, connective tissue diseases, asbestosis, lymphangitic carcinomatosis, lymphoma, lymphangioleiomyomatosis, drug-induced diseases.

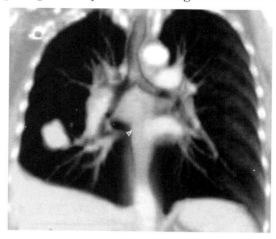

Fig. 11

Lymphadenopathy: Infections, sarcoidosis, silicosis (sarcoidosis and silicosis may be associated with lymph nodes that are calcified in an eggshell pattern), berylliosis, lymphangitic carcinomatosis, lymphoma, lymphocytic interstitial pneumonia.

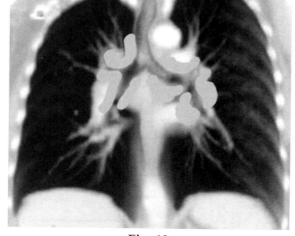

Fig. 12

In summary when evaluating a patient with diffuse lung disease

Differential diagnosis is created from the following list:
1. Type of opacity— round, linear, irregular or ground glass.
2. Location—upper, lower, diffuse.
3. Lung volume —increased, decreased, normal.
4. Ancillary finding—pneumothorax, effusion, adenopathy.
5. HRCT—septal, centrilobular, panlobular, bronchovascular.

With the above said parameters the clinical profile of the illness is kept in mind while generating a list of differentials.

See the accompanying CD for presentation on pattern approach and HRCT.

Section 3

Cases

ALLERGIC BRONCHOPULMONARY ASPERGILLOSIS (ABPA)

Definition

Allergic bronchopulmonary aspergillosis (ABPA) is a hypersensitivity disease of the lungs almost always caused by *Aspergillus fumigatus colonizing as mycelial plugs in proximal airways usually the second or third order bronchi.*

Types

1. Acute ABPA.
2. Chronic ABPA.

Incidence

- 1-2% in patients with asthma
- 10% of patients with cystic fibrosis.

Mechanism	Disease
Inhalation of conidia	*Hypersensitivity pneumonia*
Colonization	Allergic bronchopulmonary aspergillosis *Aspergilloma*
Involvement of airways	*Tracheobronchitis*
Invasion of parenchyma	Acute necrotizing aspergillus pneumonia *Lung ball* *Granulomatous aspergillosis* *Chronic necrotizing pulmonary aspergillosis*

Primary Criteria

- Asthma
- Eosinophilia
- Immediate skin test reactivity
- Precipitating antibodies (IgG)
- Elevated serum (IgE)
- Pulmonary infiltrates

CT FINDINGS

- Central varicose bronchiectasis (Fig. 1A)
- Gloved finger appearance (see case) from mucus filled airways
- High attenuation mucus plugs due to fixation of calcium and other metal ions (Fig. 1B).
- Fleeting infiltrates (migratory pneumonitis)
- Abnormalities of lung attenuation due to mosaic perfusion and air trapping.

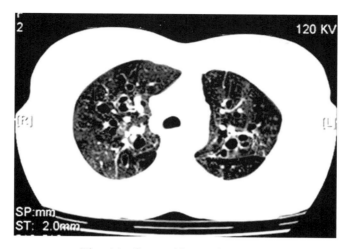

Fig. 1A: Central bronchiectasis

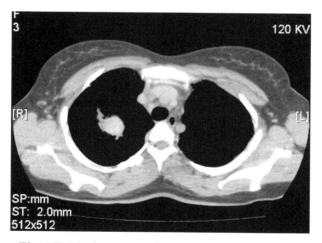

Fig. 1B: High attenuation mucus plug (arrow)

Differential Diagnosis

- Hypersensitivity pneumonitis, Loeffler's syndrome
- Consolidation, atelectasis, lobar shrinkage, pleural effusion.

ABSCESS

Definition

An inflammatory mass within lung parenchyma, the central portion of which has undergone purulent liquefaction necrosis. There may or may not be communication with the bronchial tree.

- Abscesses
  - Localized suppurative necrosis 1-6 cm
  - Right sided abscesses most often seen in aspiration pneumoniae
  - Staphylococcus; Klebsiella; Pseudomonas

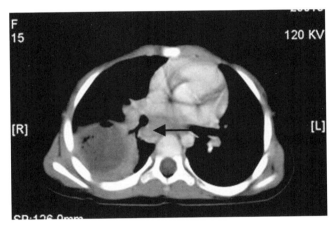

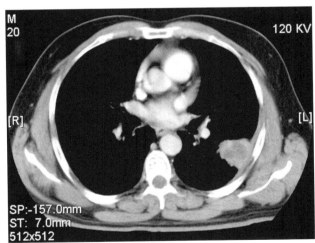

Figs 2A and B

CT FINDINGS

Abscesses present as masses in the lung, often with indistinct margins. Having low attenuation centre. If the process extends into a bronchus (arrow in 2A), the abscess contents may decompress out through the bronchus and air may move into the abscess cavity.

Differential Diagnosis

1. Infections:
    (a) Pyogenic abscess (either evolving from a necrotizing pneumonia or from aspiration).
    (b) Fungus: *Aspergillus*, *Mucor*, *Cocci*, *Crypto*, etc.
    (c) Mycobacteria
    (d) Nocardia
    (e) Parasites: *Echinococcus*, *Paragonomiasis*

Important differential diagnosis is necrotizing pneumonitis: CT appearance of necrotizing pneumonia is charecterised by multiple poorly defined foci of low density unassociated with enhancing margin of the lesion.

2. Non-infectious lesions such as:
    (a) Cavitating lung carcinoma
    (b) Metastases
    (c) Wegener's granuloma.

Complications

- Empyema.
- Secondary fungal involvement.
- Pseudoaneurysm.
- Bronchopleural fistulae.

ACINUS

Definition

The largest lung unit in which all airways participate in gas exchange is defined as a unit of lung structure distal to a terminal bronchiole. Size = 6-10 mm diameter. Supplied by a first order respiratory bronchiole.

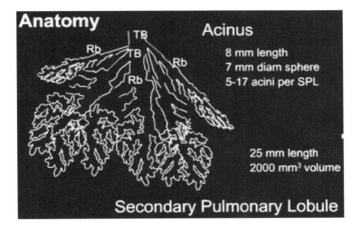

Fig. 3A

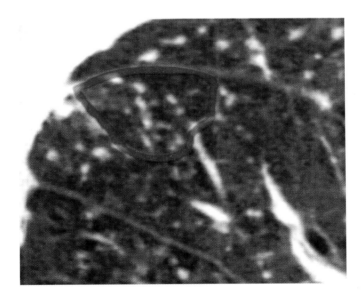

Fig. 3B

CT FINDINGS

Acinar opacity: Focal area of bronchoalveolar inflammation or air space consolidation. Presents as centrilobular ill-defined nodules measuring few mm to 1 cm in diameter (arrow).

HELPFUL HIGH-RESOLUTION CT AND TIME FACTORS IN DIFFERENTIATING ALVEOLAR FILLING DISEASES
HRCT Findings
Widely disseminated: PCP, CMV pneumonia, acute PE, ARDS, DPH, PAP, BAC, BOOP, CEP, and CSS
Localized: Segmental or peribronchial: pneumonia with *S. aureus* and *St. pyogenes*, gram-negative organisms, lipoid pneumonia, pulmonary infarction
Nonsegmental: Pneumonia with *St. pneumoniae, K. pneumoniae, Legionella* species, *M. tuberculosis*, radiation pneumonitis, BAC, and BALT lymphoma
Time Factors
Acute (within 2 weeks)
Actue pneumonia, PE, ARDS, DPH, and pulmonary infarction
Subacute or chronic (more than 1 month): Chronic pneumonia (actinomycosis, semi-invasive pulmonary aspergillosis, TB, histoplasmosis), radiation pneumonitis, PAP, lipoid pneumonia, BAC, BOOP, CEP, CSS, and BALT lymphoma
PCP = *Pneumocystic carinii* pneumonia; CMV = cytomegalovirus; PE = pulmonary edema; ARDS = adult respiratory distress syndrome; BOOP = bronchiolitis obliterans organizing pneumonia; DPH = diffuse pulmonary hemorrhage; BAC = bronchoalveolar carcinoma; TB = tuberculosis.

ADENOCARCINOMA

Definition

Mitotic lung lesion with intermediate malignant potential. Adenocarcinoma of the lung comprises 35% of lung cancer cases. The tumor is commonly peripheral in location, presenting as a solitary nodule or mass. The pathologic characteristic is glandular formations with intracellular and intraluminal mucin. Sputum cytologic examination is often negative, and bronchoscopy frequently fails to demonstrate the tumor because of the peripheral location. Scar carcinomas or bronchogenic carcinomas arising in parenchymal scars are most often adenocarcinomas. Patients with small (Stage 1) adenocarcinomas have the best prognosis after surgery of all bronchogenic carcinomas. Easy brain metastasis has been reported.

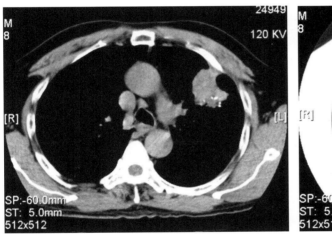 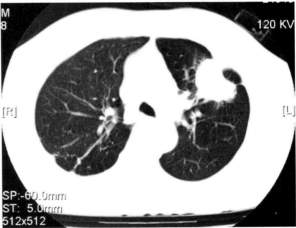

Figs 4A and B: (A) CT shows a left upper lobe peripheral mass with marginal spiculation with calcific specs. (B) Lung window showing marginal speculation around the mass (corna radiate)

CT FINDINGS

- Solitary peripheral subpleural mass
- Diameter usually less than 4 cm
- Less than 4% cavitate
- 51% show mediastinal lymphadenopathy
- Amorphous calcification may be seen in the periphery.

AIR TRAPPING

Definition

Abnormal retention of air within a lung or lung unit on expiratory scans, seen in asthma and obliterative bronchiolitis caused by partial airway obstruction.

Associations

1. Bronchiectasis
2. Mucoid impaction
3. Mucus plugs

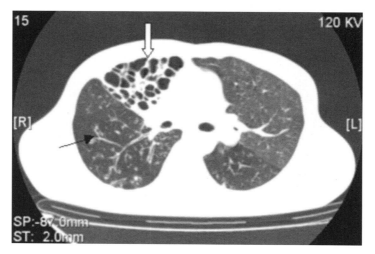

Fig. 5

CF FINDINGS

Lucent lung parenchyma with less than normal increase in attenuation seen on post-expiratory CT (arrow). There may be associated findings like mosaic attenuation, bronchiectasis (thick arrow), bronchial dilatation and mucus plugs.

Differential Diagnosis

Mosaic perfusion—Areas of decreased attenuation on inspiratory scans.
Cause: Decreased perfusion of areas distal to bronchiolar obstruction with blood flow redistribution to uninvolved lung.

ARCHITECTURAL DISTORTION

Definition

Abnormal displacement of pulmonary structures like bronchi, vessels, with distorted appearance of lung occurring due to fibrosis as a sequlae to chronic lung diseases of diverse origins.

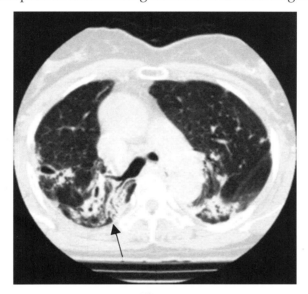

Fig. 6

CT FINDINGS

CT shows volume loss with cicatrisation causing crowding of the bronchovascular markings with fibrosis involving both lower lobes with cicatrizial bronchiectatic changes (arrow).

ASPERGILLOMA

Definition

Mass like collection of intertwined hyphae of aspergillus matted together with fibrin, mucus and cellular debris colonizing a pre-existing pulmonary cavity in immunologically normal patients. Usually seen in males over 40 years of age, presents with hemoptysis in upto 50% of patients.

Aspergillomas

Pulmonary disease caused by Aspergillus species presents with a wide spectrum of conditions. Invasive pulmonary aspergillosis is a devastating infection with a high mortality rate. The fungus itself is responsible for lung destruction. The progressive nature of the disease and its refractoriness to therapy are, in part, related to the organism's rapid growth and its tendency to invade blood vessels.

This disease is almost exclusively seen in immunocompromised hosts such as patients with (1) neutropenia, (2) bone marrow (3) or organ transplant, (4) acquired immunodeficiency.

Semi invasive or chronic necrotizing aspergillosis is an indolent, destructive process of lung, seen in middle-aged or elderly patients with lung disease like COPD, TB, pneumoconiosis, patients with mild immunosuppression. It is an indolent process continuing over months/years.

Predisposing Pulmonary Conditions associated with Development of Aspergilloma

- Tuberculosis cavity
- Cavitary neoplasm
- Pulmonary fibrosis
- Radiation fibrosis
- Lung abscess
- Bronchial cyst
- Asbestosis
- Histoplasmosis
- Blastomycosis
- Ankylosing spondylitis
- Bronchiectasis
- Pneumonia
- Cyanotic heart disease
- Pulmonary infarction
- Invasive aspergillosis
- ABPA
- HIV infection.

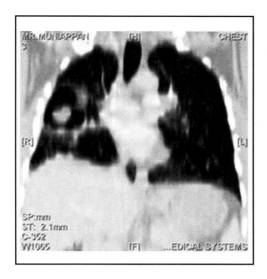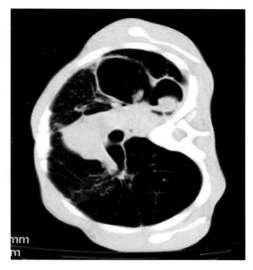

Figs 7A and B

CT FINDINGS

Aspergilloma:

Mounod sign— Solid round gravity dependent mass within pre-existing spherical/ovoid thin walled cavity

Air crescent separates fungus ball from cavity wall.

Scattered/rim-like calcification of fungus ball.

Enhancement of wall of cavity due to hypertrophy of supplying bronchial arteries.

Adjacent pleural thickening.

Cavity may be due to tuberculosis, sarcoidosis, bronchiectasis, bulla or carcinoma.

Differential Diagnosis of Aspergilloma

* Cavitating neoplasm
* Blood clot in pulmonary cavity
* Hydatid cyst (disintegrating)
* Pulmonary abscess with necrosis
* Non-Aspergillus spp mycetoma.

Semi invasive

* Parenchymal consolidative changes.
* May have cavitary changes.
* No features of invasion.

Invasive (also see Case 38, Fig. 38B)

* Multiple nodules, with zone of low attenuation due to hemorrhage, so called halosign.
* Consolidative changes reflecting infarcts.

ASTHMA

A disease characterized by widespread reversible narrowing of the bronchial airways, changing rapidly in severity either spontaneously or with treatment.

The chest X-ray is normal in most patients with bronchial asthma, and what radiographic findings are seen don't correlate well with the severity of an attack. In severe cases, one may see X-ray evidence of severe overinflation and air trapping (flattened diaphragmatic domes, increased retrosternal air space).

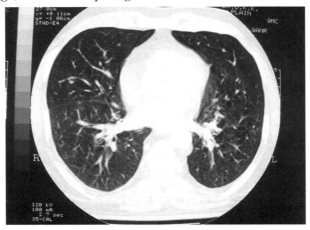

Fig. 8

CT FINDINGS

- Peribronchial cuffing
- Bronchial dilatation
- Localized areas of hypoattenuation
- Mucoid impaction
- Chronic cases-bronchiectasis, scars

Complications—Pneumonia, atelectasis, pneumothorax, pneumomediastinum, emphysema, allergic bronchopulmonary aspergillosis.

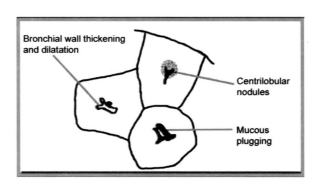

Fig. 8A

ATELECTASIS

Definition

Loss of inflation of all or a portion of the lung, with corresponding diminution of lung volume. Based on distribution classified as lobar, subsegmental, plate-like, etc.

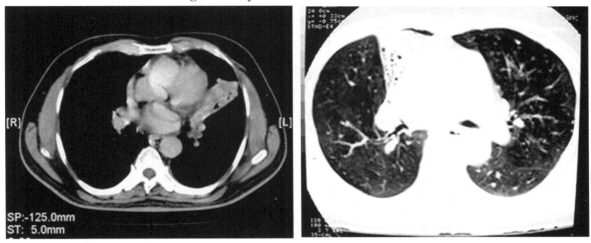

Figs 9A and B: (A) Left lingular resorptive atelectasis. (B) Right middle lobe cicatrizial atelectasis

The only direct sign is displacement of an interlobar fissure.

Indirect signs include a local increase in opacity, elevation of a hemidiaphragm, mediastinal displacement, compensatory overinflation of other lung segments, displacement of the hila, changes in the chest wall, and absence of an air bronchogram.

CT Findings

The CT findings include:
1. Irregular narrowing or occlusion of the airway.
2. Involved lobe appears wedge shaped with a 'V' shape.
3. Large tumor masses produce a bulge in the contour of the collapsed lobe called golden s sign.
4. Rarely entire lobe may be replaced by a tumor without a bronchial obstruction.

CAUSES

LARGE AIRWAY OBSTRUCTION
- LUMINAL
  - Primary tumor (carcinoma, carcinoid, etc.)
  - Secondary tumor (kidney, breast, thyroid)
  - Endobronchial granuloma (TB, sarcoid)
  - Foreign body (including wrongly placed ET tube)
- MURAL
  - Inflammatory stricture (TB)
  - Bronchial atresia

- Bronchial rupture, transection
- Sarcoidosis
- Wegener's granulomatosis
- Amyloidosis
- EXTRAMURAL
  - Adenopathy (inflammatory/neoplastic)
  - Mediastinal masses
  - Cardiomegaly (enlarged LA)
  - Aneurysms and vascular malformations
  - Fibrosing mediastinitis

SMALL AIRWAY OBSTRUCTION

- MUCUS PLUGS
  - Cystic fibrosis
  - Asthma
  - Postoperative patient
  - Respiratory depressant drugs (morphine)
- INFLAMMATORY
  - Bronchopneumonia
  - Bronchitis
  - Bronchiectasis

TYPES OF ATELECTASIS

COMPRESSIVE ATELECTASIS

- Peripheral tumor
- Extensive interstitial disease (sarcoidosis, lymphoma)
- Air trapping in adjacent lung (bullous emphysema, foreign body obstruction)

PASSIVE ATELECTASIS

- Pneumothorax
- Hydrothorax
- Diaphragmatic hernia
- Pleural mass (mesothelioma, metastasis)

ADHESIVE ATELECTASIS

- Respiratory distress syndrome of newborn
- Pulmonary embolism

CICATRIZATION ATELECTASIS

- Tuberculosis
- Scleroderma
- Silicosis
- Histoplasmosis
- Idiopathic pulmonary fibrosis
- Radiation pneumonitis (chronic phase)

AZYGOUS LOBE FISSURE

Part of the apical or posterior segments of the right upper lobe laterally limited by the azygous fissure. They have a incidence of 4% in the general population. The fissures have 4 layers of pleura (2 parietal, 2 visceral).

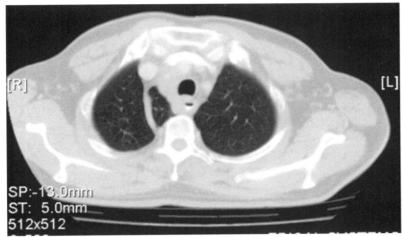

Fig. 10

CT FINDINGS

Azygous fissure is seen as a thin curved line extending from the right brachiocephalic vein anteriorly to the right superior intercostal vein.

ACCESSORY FISSURES

Accessory fissures are clefts of varying depths in the outer surface of the lung that delineates accessory lobe. Six important accessory fissures are recognized

1. Azygous fissure.
2. Inferior accessory fissure—separates medial basal from rest of the lower lobe segments.
3. Superior accessory fissure—separates apical segment of lower lobe from basal segments.
4. Inferior pulmonary ligament—sheet of pleura hangs down from hilum, joins the lung to the mediastinum and to medial part of diaphragm.
5. Left minor fissure—rare (8%) separates lingual from upper lobe.
6. Left azygous fissure—involves left hemiazygous vein.

ALVEOLAR PROTEINOSIS

Infiltrative lung disease in which air spaces are filled with PAS positive lipoproteinaceous material. May be idiopathic or secondary to other causes like dust exposure. Males, age-30 to 50 years. Chest X-ray—Bilateral perihilar patchy or diffuse consolidation, especially at lung bases.

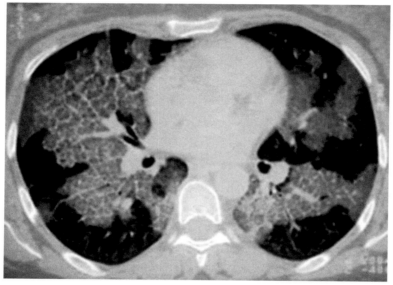

Fig. 11

CT FINDINGS

Crazy paving appearance—Bilateral areas of geographically distributed ground glass attenuation with associated interlobular septal thickening.

Differential Diagnosis

Acute—Focal pneumonia, pulmonary edema, ARDS. Chronic-idiopathic pulmonary hemosiderosis, Goodpasture's syndrome, hypersensitivity pneumonitis, desquamative interstitial pneumonia.

ACUTE RESPIRATORY DISTRESS SYNDROME (ARDS)

Severe life-threatening acute respiratory distress with abrupt onset of dyspnea, hypoxemia associated with widespread air space consolidation.

Predisposing conditions—shock, infections, drugs, drowning, trauma.

Direct Lung Injury (Pulmonary ARDS)	Indirect Lung Injury (Extrapulmonary ARDS)
Aspiration	Sepsis
Diffuse pulmonary infection • Bacterial • Viral • Protozoal	Severe non-thoracic trauma
Near drowning	Hypertransfusion (during emergency resuscitation)
Toxic fume inhalation	Cardiopulmonary bypass (rare)
Lung contusion	

Stages and Findings

	Histopathology	CXR	CT scan
1	• Capillary congestion • Endothelial swelling • Exudation of inflammatory fluid into interstitium • Minimal fluid in alveoli	• Normal	
2	• Sloughing of epithelial lining of alveolar cells • Flooding of airspaces	• Homogenous ground glass appearance	• Heterogeneous ground glass appearance • Bronchial dilatation
3	• Alveolar atelectasis • Hyaline membrane formation	• Homogenous ground glass with possible consolidation in dependent areas	• Heterogeneous ground glass with possible consolidation in dependent areas-Bronchial dilatation
4	• Proliferation of fibroblasts and type II pneumocytes-extensive consolidation in alveoli	"	"
5	• Chronic phase: type II pneumocyte hyperplasia and collagen deposition • Resolves lung tissue to normal or becomes interstitial fibrosis	• Resolves to normal or coarse reticular opacities	• Resolves or get a reticular pattern, commonly in ventral non-dependent lung

Differential Diagnosis

- Pulmonary edema
- Granulomatous disease
- Infection
- IPF
- Pneumoconiosis
- Drug toxicity
- Tumor

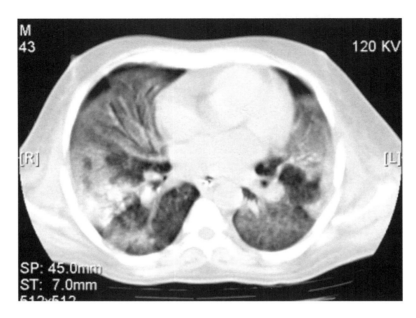

Fig. 12A: Acute bilateral airspace opacity

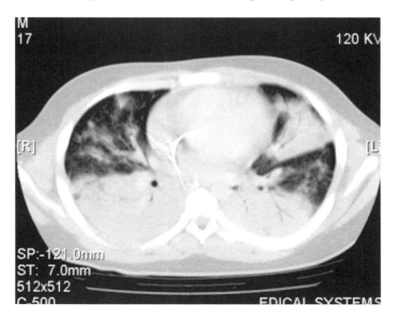

Fig. 12B: Plain CT shows bilateral multifocal parenchymal consolidation

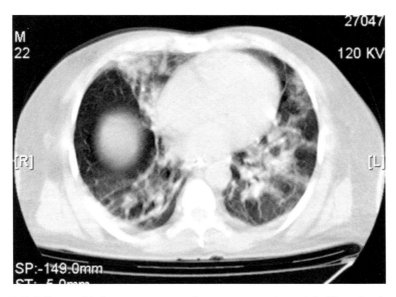

Fig. 12C: Bilateral inhomogenous air space opacity with fibrotic changes

CT FINDINGS

1st day—patchy ill-defined bilateral parenchymal opacities (Fig. 12A).
2nd day—massive bilateral consolidation, predominant at lung bases.
1st week—inhomogenous consolidation (Fig. 12B)
>1week—reticular pattern due to fibrosis with or without large subpleural cysts (Fig. 12C).

CASE 13

ASPIRATION

Aspiration pneumoniae refers to the pulmonary consequences resulting from the abnormal entry of fluid, particulate exogenous /endogenous substances. Aspiration of gastric contents occur in women during parturition, called as Mendelson syndrome, other causes include aspiration in patients with altered sensorium. Dysphagia from neurologic deficits, esophageal disease, tracheostomy, most pneumonias arise from microorganism in the oral cavity or nasopharynx (streptococcus, haemophilus, staphylococcus).

Clinically characterized by acute onset cyanosis, dyspnea, tachypnea, pathologically characterized by chemical tracheobronchitis, with pneumonia, abscess formation, ARDS or even pulmonary embolism.

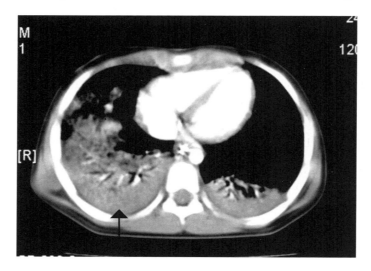

Fig. 13

CT FINDINGS

CT is characterized by diffuse bibasilar alveolar consolidation (arrow). In uncomplicated cases there is clearing of alveolar shadows in 4-6 days.

Persistent radiographic worsening is a cause for concern and patient has to be evaluated for ARDS, bacterial pneumonia, and bacterial infection.

BRONCHIOLITIS

Definition—Generic term used to describe bronchiolar inflammation of various causes. They are classified into two groups:
1. Those resulting from thickening of the bronchiolar walls.
2. Those resulting from obstruction to bronchiolor lumen.

Indicates an idiopathic syndrome of chronic airflow obstruction in patients without underlying emphysema or chronic bronchitis.

Dilated bronchioles, which when fluid filled give tree-in-bud appearance.

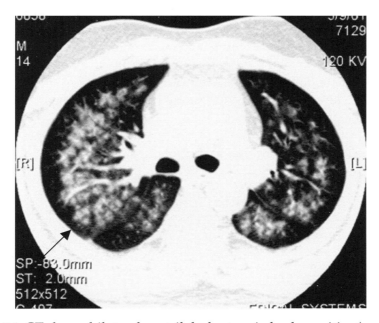

Fig. 14: CT shows bilateral centrilobular tree in bud opacities (arrow)

Pathologically classified into:
1. Cellular bronchiolitis
2. Panbronchiolitis.
3. Respiratory bronchiolitis.
4. Constrictive bronchiolitis.
5. BOOP.

Depending on CT appearance, bronchiolar disease is classified as follows:
1. Bronchiolar disease with tree-in-bud pattern
   Diffuse panbronchiolitis
   Infectious bronchiolitis- especially endobronchial tuberculosis.

Tree-in-bud refers to dilated mucus filled terminal and respiratory bronchioles resulting in centrilobular nodular, branching, or Y-shaped densities. Seen in lung periphery

2. Bronchiolar disease with poorly defined centrilobular nodules
   Sub-acute hypersensitivity pneumonitis
   Lymphoid interstitial pneumonia.
   Follicular bronchiolitis
   Respiratory bronchiolitis- ILD
   Mineral dust induced bronchiolitis
   Characterized by ill-defined centrilobular nodules in the absence of tree-in-bud appearance and consolidation
   Pathologically correlate- peribronchiolar inflammation without dilatation or retained secretions
3. Bronchiolar disease associated with ground-glass attenuation and consolidation
   (BOOP) (see Case 22)
   Characterized by 1-3 month history of non-productive cough, low-grade fever and increasing shortness of breath
   Pathology—granulation tissue polyps within respiratory bronchioles and alveolar ducts with patchy organizing pneumonia
   Plain X-ray- patchy, non-segmental unilateral or bilateral foci of air space consolidation
   CT- patchy bilateral consolidation with predominantly peribronchial and subpleural distribution
4. Bronchiolar diseases associated with decreased lung attenuation
   Obliterative (constrictive) bronchiolitis (Swyer-James syndrome)—causes-heart-lung transplant, chronic rejection, collagen vascular disease
   Pathology—concentric fibrosis with narrowing of terminal and respiratory bronchioles
   HRCT—mosaic attenuation, air trapping and bronchial dilatation.

CASE 15

BRONCHIOLECTASIS

Dilated terminal bronchioles secondary to peribronchiolar fibrosis, usually seen in panbronchiolitis secondary to viral or bacterial infections. Thickened peripheral bronchioles because of their small size may appear as nodules.

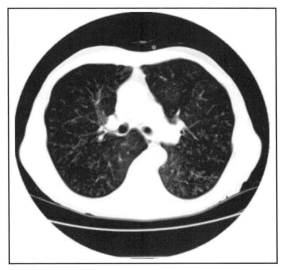

Fig. 15

CT FINDINGS

CT findings are that of multiple peripheral nodules, if the distal airways are dilated they appear as small cavitations.

CASE 16

BRONCHOLITHIASIS

It implies calcified material in the airway, including the effects of airway distortion or inflammation caused by calcified peribronchial nodes resulting in collapse, obstructive pneumonitis, mucoid obstruction. Symptoms commonly include cough, hemoptysis, recurrent fever. Commonly seen as a sequlae to tuberculosis, silicosis, cryptococcosis. Other causes include:

1. Aspiration of bone tissue or in situ calcification of aspirated foreign material.
2. Endobronchial tumor calcification.
3. Primary endobronchial infection with calcification.

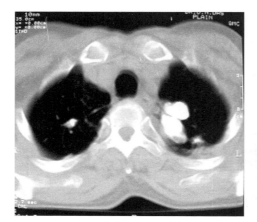 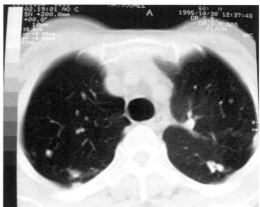

Figs 16A and B

CT FINDINGS

CT findings include calcified nodes, and endobronchial calcifications. This appearance can be mimicked by calcified endobronchial mitotic lesions or carcinoid tumors.

BRONCHOPLEURAL FISTULA

It is characterized by a communication between the bronchial system/lung parenchyma and pleural space. It differs from pneumothorax in that the communication with the pleural space is via airways rather than distal air spaces.

Commonly seen as a complication of resectional surgery like pneumonectomy/lobectomy. Blunt or penetrating trauma, barotraumas, lung necrosis due to necrotizing pneumonias.

Airway diseases like bronchiectasis, emphysema complicated by pneumonia, tuberculosis with sequlae, necrotizing malignancy.

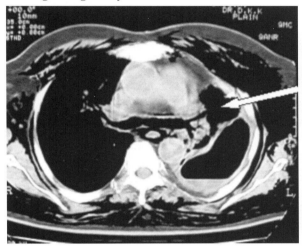

Fig. 17A

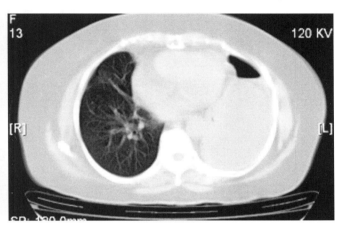

Fig. 17B: Plain CT lung showing features of empyema with airfluid level due to a peripheral bronchopleural fistula

CT FINDINGS

CT findings include demonstrating the direct communication of the fistula (arrow in Fig. 17A), peripheral persistent air fluid level with or without features of chronic empyema.

Other Features

- Lenticular in shape
- Unequal length of air fluid level in different projections.
- Split pleura seen
- Contiguous with the chest wall atleast in one projection.

BRONCHIECTASIS

Localized or diffuse irreversible dilatation of bronchi, secondary to infection, airway obstruction, inherited abnormalities, or fibrosis.

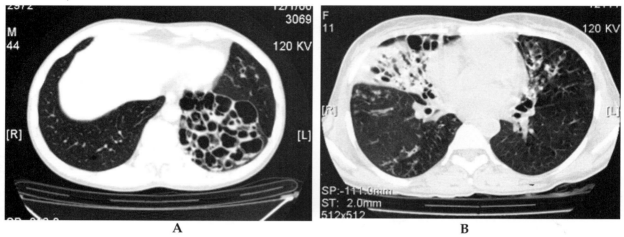

Figs 18A and B: (A) Cystic bronchiectasis in left lower lobe. (B) Cylindrical brochiectasis right middle and left lingular segments due to infective process

CONDITIONS PREDISPOSING TO BRONCHIECTASIS

Severe Inflammation

Infection

- *Mycobacterium* species (e.g. *tuberculosis, avium intracellulare*)
- Bacterial (e.g. *Staphylococcus aureus, Bordetella pertussis*)
- Viral (e.g. measles, influenza, rubeola, adenovirus, HIV)
- Fungal (e.g. histoplasmosis, coccidioidomycosis)

Hypersensitivity

- Allergic bronchopulmonary aspergillosis

Inhalation Injury

- Smoke
- Sulfur dioxide
- Ammonia

Other

- Recurrent gastric aspiration
- Heroin overdose
- Autoimmune disease (e.g. relapsing polychondritis, Behçet's syndrome)
- Diffuse panbronchiolitis.

Congenital Syndromes

- Cystic fibrosis
- Alpha1-antitrypsin deficiency
- Primary ciliary dyskinesia
  - Kartagener's syndrome (situs inversus, sinusitis, and bronchiectasis)
- Immunodeficiency states (e.g. hypogammaglobulinemia)
- Young's syndrome (azoospermia and chronic sinopulmonary infections)
- Yellow-nail syndrome (lymphedema, pleural effusions, hypertrophic nails)

Airway Obstruction

- Foreign body
- Bronchial stricture
- Airway neoplasia or nodule
  - Bronchogenic carcinoma
  - Bronchial adenoma
  - Carcinoid
  - Sarcoidosis
  - Amyloidosis
  - Broncholith
- External compression of bronchus
  - Mediastinal mass or lymph node
  - Lung cancer
  - Vascular aneurysm
  - Mediastinal fibrosis

Traction

- Pulmonary fibrosis
- Tuberculosis
- Collagen vascular disease
- Sarcoidosis
- Radiation

Anatomic Malformations or Variants

- Bronchomalacia
- Bronchial cartilage deficiency (Williams-Campbell syndrome)
- Tracheobronchomegaly (Mounier-Kuhn syndrome)
- Unilateral hyperlucent lung (Swyer-James syndrome)
- Bronchopulmonary sequestration
- Middle lobe syndrome

CLASSIFICATION

1. Cylindrical/tubular/fusiform bronchiectasis
2. Saccular/cystic bronchiectasis

3. Varicose bronchiectasis
   - Bronchial dilatation
     - "Signet ring" (cross-section of dilated bronchus + branch of pulmonary artery)
     - "Tram lines" (when the bronchi are horizontally oriented)
     - Lack of tapering
     - "String of pearls" (varicose bronchiectasis)
     - "String of cysts/cluster of cysts"
   - Bronchial wall thickening
   - Mucus/fluid retention in bronchial lumen
- Air-fluid level

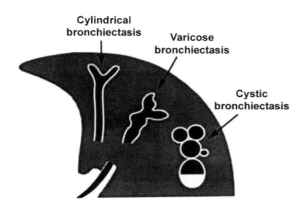

Fig. 18C: Schematic

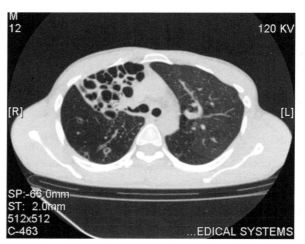

Fig. 18D: Right upper lobe cavitary bronchiectasis

BULLA

Bulla is defined as a emphysematous space within the lung with a diameter more than 1 cm. Bulla may be single or multiple.

Bulla Reid Classification of Bullae

- Type I   Subpleural, medial upper lobe, narrow neck
- Type II   Subpleural exaggeration of emphysema
- Type III   Parenchymal exaggeration of emphysema

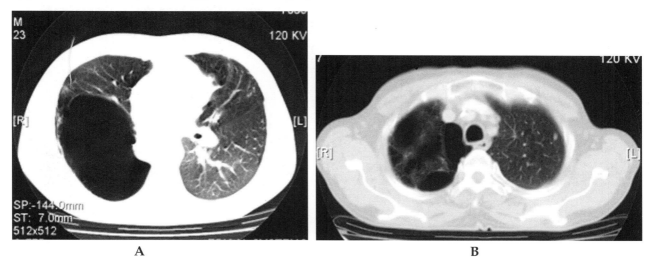

Figs 19A and B: (A) CT findings are a well-defined transradient air lucency measuring >1 cm in diameter and with wall-thickness < 1 mm in the right lower lobe. (B) Axial CT shows a grossly emphysematous left upperlobe with extensive subpleural type 2 bullous change

CT FINDINGS

CT findings are a well-defined transradiant air lucency measuring >1 cm in diameter and with wall-thickness < 1 mm in the right lower lobe.

Differential Diagnosis—Lung Cyst

Differentiating factor—Bulla is always associated with extensive emphysema.
Main complication of bullae are infection, hemorrhage, pneumothorax.
*Also see Appendix for differential diagnosis.

BUBBLE LUCENCIES

Bubble-like lucencies may be seen in adenocarcinoma, bronchoalveolar carcinoma, and pulmonary infarcts. In adenocarcinoma and bronchoalveolar carcinoma, the lucencies represent patent small airways. In pulmonary infarction, the lucencies represent aerated acini or lobules within the hemorrhagic lung.

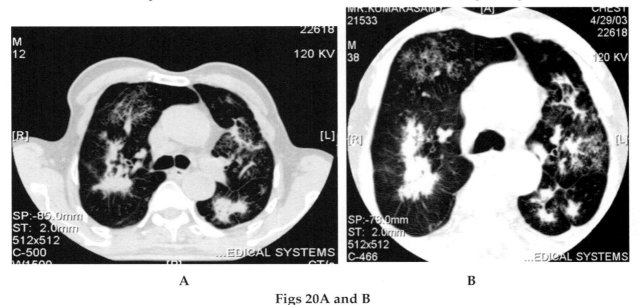

A   B

Figs 20A and B

CT FINDINGS

CT findings show bilateral multifocal parenchymal opacity with irregular margins, with lucencies within histopathology was suggestive of bronchoalveolar carcinoma.

CASE 21

BRONCHOALVEOLAR CARCINOMA

Bronchoalveolar carcinoma is characterized pathologically by lepidic growth with preservation of lung architecture. The most frequent symptoms and signs in patients with bronchoalveolar carcinoma include cough, sputum, shortness of breath, weight loss, hemoptysis, and fever. Bronchorrhea, once considered the clinical hallmark of this disease, is unusual and a late manifestation seen only with diffuse bronchoalveolar carcinoma.

The radiologic manifestations of bronchoalveolar carcinoma are diverse and include single or multiple pulmonary nodules, segmental or lobar consolidation, and diffuse air space The lobar consolidative form accounts for approximately 30% of all bronchoalveolar carcinomas and corresponds to a mucinous histologic type. The air space consolidation is caused by growth along the alveolar wall combined with secretion of mucin. Production of copious amounts of mucin may result in expansion of the involved lobe, leading to bulging of interlobar fissures.

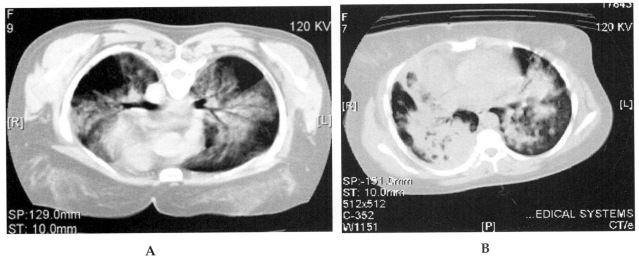

A   B

Figs 21A and B: Axial CT shows bilateral confluent alveolar opacity. Biopsy suggestive of bronchoalveolar carcinoma

CT FINDINGS

CT findings show bilateral multifocal parenchymal lobar consolidation. Prone CT was done to rule out gravity dependent summation, and for biopsy localization. HPE was suggestive of bronchoalveolar carcinoma.

BOOP

BOOP is defined as bronchiolitis obliterans organizing pneumonia characterized histologically by granulation tissue polyps also called mason bodies in the bronchiolar and peribronchiolar regions.

BOOP Pathology Not Specific	
Collagen vascular diseases	Rheumatoid arthritis Systemic lupus erythematosus Dermatomyositis Mixed connective tissue disease
Toxins	Inhalants (crack cocaine, NO_2) Drugs (bleomycin, amiodarone)
Chronic infection	Bacteria (Legionella, Nocardia) Viruses (AIDS, CMV, *Influenza*) *Mycoplasma* *Pneumocystis carinii*
Idiopathic	Cryptogenic organizing pneumonia

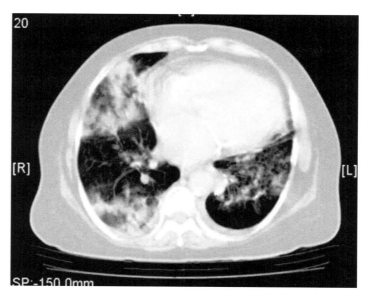

Fig. 22: Axial HRCT reveals bilateral multisegmental peripheral consolidations

Clinical Features

- Middle aged adults (40 - 60 years old)
- Subacute
  - May be fulminant with progression to respiratory failure and ARDS
- Gradual onset of dyspnea, dry cough and low-grade fever
  - Systemic symptoms
- Restrictive pulmonary function

CT FINDINGS

- Bilateral consolidation/ground-glass
  - Air bronchograms
- All lung zones involved
- Subpleural distribution
- Nodules 1-10 mm in size
- Adenopathy, pleural effusion may be noted

BRONCHOGENIC CYST

- Pathophysiology—anomalous bud from tracheobronchial tree between 5th-16th week gestation
  - Arrested in embryonic stage
  - Contain tissue normally found in trachea/bronchi
    - mucus glands
    - smooth muscle
    - elastic tissue
    - cartilage
  - Can enlarge due to secretion production, become fluid-filled
- Location—
  - paratracheal
  - carinal
  - paraesophageal
  - hilar

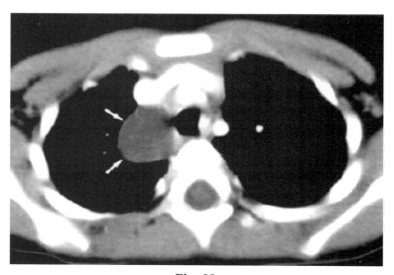

Fig. 23

CT FINDINGS

CT findings show a well marginated hypodense lesion in the right paratracheal region with smooth contour.

- Clinical manifestations—result from compression of adjacent structures
  - cough
  - stridor
  - wheezing
  - air trapping and obstructive emphysema, mediastinal shift
  - atelectasis
  - impaired secretion clearance if recurrent pneumonia
  - dysphagia, epigastric discomfort, chest pain, etc.
  - symptom can develop at any age (5-19% are asymptomatic)

- typically presents with airway compression and respiratory distress in infancy presents in childhood due to retained secretions and infection
- smooth contoured mass
- may have air-fluid level

Bronchopulmonary Foregut Malformations can be classified as:

- Ventral budding from the foregut or tracheobronchial tree
  - Sequestration
  - Bronchogenic cyst
- Sequestration—Induction of mesenchymal development into lung parenchymal
- Bronchogenic cyst—Failure to induce mesenchymal development into lung parenchyma

BRONCHIAL ATRESIA

Bronchial atresia is a pulmonary anomaly of unknown etiology in which a segmental bronchi does not communicate with the central airways.

Pathogenesis

- Sequlae of a vascular insult to the lung parenchyma during early fetal development (15-16 weeks).
- Occurs secondary to separation of the bronchial bud during 5-6th week of gestation.
- Most of the cases are asymptomatic and are incidental findings on radiographs.

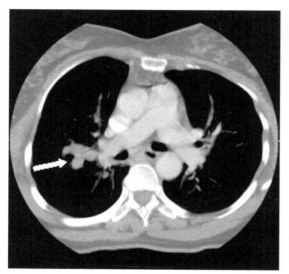
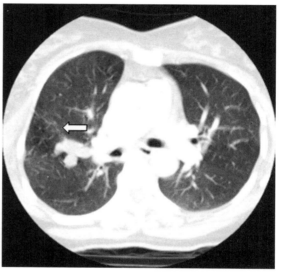

| A | B |

Figs 24A and B: Axial CT in mediastinal window shows linear, tubular structure at the level of hilum, showing low attenuation centre (arrow in Fig. 24A), adjacent lung shows transradiancy (arrow in Fig. 24B)

CT FINDINGS

1. Finger like opacity lateral to hilum (mucous plug distal to atretic lumen).
2. Expanded segment (collateral air drift with expiratory air-trapping).

Differential Diagnosis

Congenital lobar emphysema (no mucous plug).

CAVITY

An abnormal pulmonary parenchymal space, not containing lung but filled with air and/or fluid, created by tissue necrosis, with a defined wall at least 1 mm in thickness, lined with neoplastic and/or inflammatory elements.

Mechanism: Tissue necrosis with subsequent communication with the tracheobronchial tree.

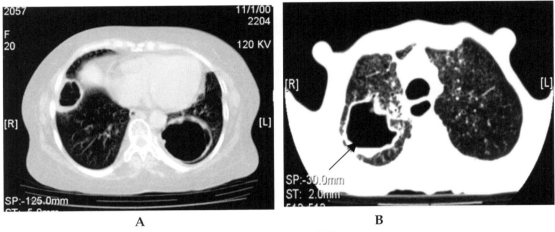

A   B

Figs 25A and B

CT FINDINGS

CT findings are of a well marginated lucent parenchymal zones, with variable wall thickness.
A. Bilateral well marginated cavitary lesions involving the right lower zone anteriorly, and left lower zone posteriorly.
B. Right upper lobe cavity with adjacent parenchymal nodular opacities suggestive of a Koch's lesion with transbronchial spread (arrow).

Pulmonary Lucency: Radiographic Approach

a. Single vs multiple
b. Distribution: upper vs lower, central vs peripheral, dependent distribution (superior segments lower lobes, apical and posterior segments of upper lobes).
c. Wall thickness
d. Character of wall
e. Inner contents:
   1. Air/fluid levels
   2. Internal opacities (mobile or not)
f. Associated findings:
   1. Pleural effusions
   2. Adenopathy
   3. Nodules
   4. Air space disease
   5. Chest wall abnormalities
g. Patient demographics and clinical history.

CONGLOMERATE MASS (PROGRESSIVE MASSIVE FIBROSIS)

A large opacity, representing a mass of fibrous tissue, seen surrounding and encompassing bronchi and vessels in the central/parahilar lung.

Seen in
1. Sarcoidosis
2. Silicosis
3. CWP
4. Tuberculosis
5. IV drug abusers with talcosis

Differences in CT Findings Between Conglomerate Masses in Sarcoidosis and Pneumoconiosis		
Features	*Sarcoidosis*	*Pneumoconiosis*
Area of lung	Upper lobes	Upper lobes
Appearance	Irregular with peripheral discrete nodules, encompassing bronchioles which are dilated and crowded together	Homogenous opacity
Traction bronchiectasis	Associated	Not associated
Adjacent emphysema	Absent	Present

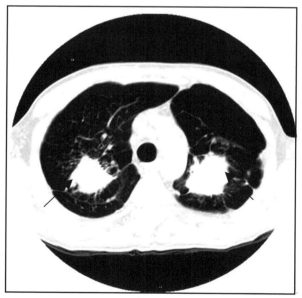

Fig. 26

CT FINDINGS

CT findings show bilateral upper zone parenchymal mass lesion (arrows) with adjacent parenchymal cicatrizial changes. Patient was a known case of silicosis on follow-up.

CASE 27

CONSOLIDATION

Area of increased opacity in the lung with obscuration of underlying vessels. Indicates replacement of alveolar air by fluid, cells or other material.

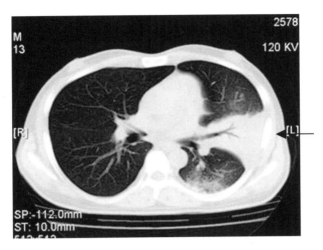

Fig. 27A

CT FINDINGS

CT findings show left mid zone segmental parenchymal consolidation with air bronchogram (arrow).
- Common organisms
  - *Streptococcus pneumoniae*
  - *Haemophilus influenzae*
  - Legionella
  - Pseudomonas sp.

FOUR STAGES

- Stage 1 : Congestion
  Boggy engorged alveolar vessels
- Stage 2: Red hepatization
  Lobe is confluently filled with intra-alveolar PMNs and RBCs resulting in a 'liver-like' state
- Stage 3: Gray hepatization
  Lobe pales as PMNs ingest and destroy RBCs, other inflammatory debris and bacteria
- Stage 4: Resolution

Four basic pattern of infective pneumonia include:
- Bronchopneumonia- multifocal filling of airways.
- Spherical —ill-defined round areas of consolidation.
- Interstitial— widespread peribronchial thickening with ill-defined reticular shadows.

PATTERN OF INVOLVEMENT

1. Lobar/segmental—bacterial, atypical
2. Expanding lobar—Staph., gram negatives, *Klebsiella*, anaerobes
3. Cavitating—Staph., gram negatives, *Klebsiella*, anaerobes, fungi
4. Generalized alveolar—bacterial, pneumocystis
5. Generalized interstitial—viral, TB, atypical, fungal, pneumocystis
6. Crescentic—hydatid, fungal
7. Effusion—bacterial, TB
8. Extrapulmonary—actinomycosis, hydatid
9. Pneumothorax—Staphylococci, *Klebsiella*
10. Lymphadenopathy—viral, TB, fungal, actinomycosis.

Expected time for resolution of pneumonia due to common respiratory pathogens		
Pathogen	*Typical time required for radiographic clearing*	*Frequency of scarring, residual lesions*
Streptococcus pneumoniae (nonbacteremic)	1-3 mo	Rare
Mycoplasma pneumoniae	2 wk-2 mo	Rare
Chlamydia species	1-3 mo	Infrequent
Legionella species	2-6 mo	10%-25%
Staphylococcus aureus	3-5 mo	Frequent
Enteric gram-negative bacilli	3-5 mo	Frequent
Viruses	Unknown	Varicella pneumonia: diffuse punctate calcifications; atypical measles: nodules

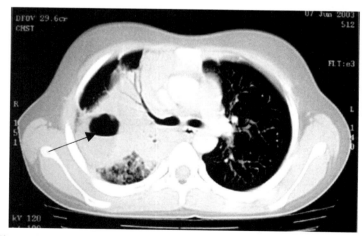

Fig. 27B: Axial CT shows a cavitary pneumonia with a air fluid level suggestive or a evolving abscess (arrow)

CYST

The term *cyst* is nonspecific and refers to a thin-walled (usually less than 3 mm thick), well-defined and circumscribed, air- or fluid-containing lesion, 1 cm or more in diameter, that has an epithelial or fibrous wall. A cystic pattern results from a heterogeneous group of diseases, all having in common the presence of focal, multifocal, or diffuse parenchymal lucencies and lung destruction

Differential Diagnosis

Pulmonary Langerhans' cell histiocytosis, lymphangioleiomyomatosis, sarcoidosis, lymphocytic interstitial pneumonitis, *Pneumocystis carinii* pneumonia, honeycombing, and centrilobular emphysema can manifest a cystic pattern on **HRCT**.

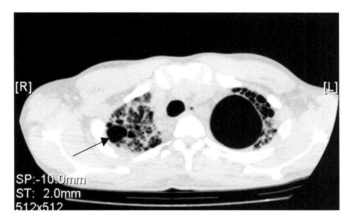

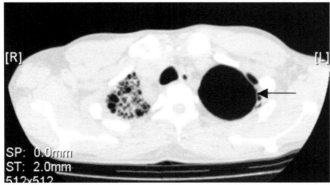

Figs 28A and B

CT FINDINGS

CT findings in a paitent with end stage interstitial pneumonia showing multiple lucent spaces with conglomeration reflecting gross honeycombing with cyst formation (arrow).

CASE 29

COMPENSATORY HYPERINFLATION

Compensatory changes seen in a lobe or lung due to diseases process in the adjacent lung zones.

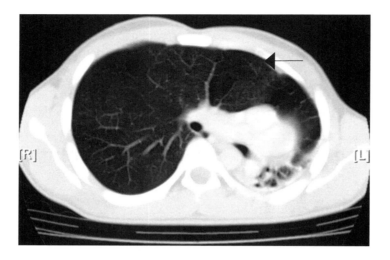

Fig. 29

CT FINDINGS

CT findings include increase in right lung volume, with increased translucency and substernal herniation to the contralateral side (arrow). The pathological lung on left shows end stage cystic changes/cicatricial fibrosis.

CASE 30

CYSTIC FIBROSIS

Definition—Autosomal recessive multisystem disease characterized by mucous plugging of exocrine glands secondary to formation of thick tenacious secretions and defective mucociliary transport:

- Age—almost all cases diagnosed by 12 years of age
- No sex predeliction
- Elevated concentration of sodium and chloride in sweat
- Increased susceptibility for infection with pseudomonas and staphylococcus
- Characterized by chronic cough with recurrent respiratory infections
- Predeliction for apical and posterior segments of upper lobes

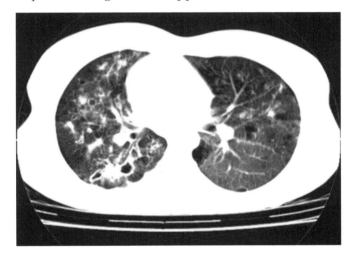

Fig. 30: Axial HRCT reveals right lower lobe and middle lobe impacted bronchi with bronchiectatic cyst. Left lingula shows hyperinflation

CT FINDINGS

- Cylindrical/cystic bronchiectasis
- Finger-like mucus plugs
- Peribronchial thickening
- Bronchiectatic cyst—bronchus directly leading to sacculation
- Emphysematous bullae
- Paraseptal emphysema
- Subsegmental/segmental collapse with RUL predominance
- Areas of consolidation may be associated

Complications

- Recurrent infections
- ABPA
- Cor pulmonale and pulmonary hypertension
- Hemoptysis
- Pneumothorax
- Hypertrophic pulmonary osteoarthropathy

CASE 31

CHRONIC EOSINOPHILIC PNEUMONIA (CEP)

CEP is an idiopathic condition characterized by filling in of air spaces. With eosinophils and macrophages associated with interstitial pneumonia.

    Seen in middle age women with peripheral eosinophilia.

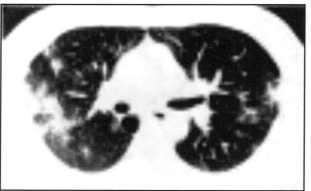 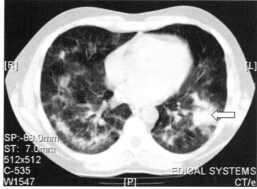

Fig. 31

CT FINDINGS

CT scan shows subpleural areas of consolidation in the right and left mid zones (arrow in Fig. 31B). In the early stage of the disease, consolidation is the predominant abnormality on CT, described as photographic negative of pulmonary edema, whereas nodules or reticular densities predominate in later stages.

CLINICAL FEATURES OF EOSINOPHILIC PNEUMONIAS				
	Chronic eosinophilic pneumonia	Acute eosinophilic pneumonia	Löffler's syndrome	Tropical eosinophilia
Blood eosinophilia	X		X	X
Transitory patchy pulmonary infiltrates	X		X	
Elevated IgE			X	X
Infiltrates	X	X	X	X
Occurs in middle-aged asthmatic women	X			
Alveolar filling	X	X		
BAL fluid eosinophils		X		
ELISA positive for filarial antibodies				X
Cough, wheeze, dyspnea, etc.	X		X	X
Steroid responsive	X	X	X	X
Resolves spontaneously			X	
Recurs	X			

CASE 32

CONGENITAL LOBAR EMPHYSEMA

Its thought to be a sequlae to an yet unidentified cause of dysplasia of the bronchial support structures. Definite association with congenital heart disease present.

Usually presents as neonatal respiratory distress.

Seen on chest X-ray as a hyperexpansion of an upper or middle lobe, the expanded lung may cause compression atelectasis of the adjacent lobes.

CT FEATURES

- Lobar hyperinflation with compression of adjacent atelectatic lung
- May be initially opaque mimicking a solid lesion
- Mass effect, mediastinal shift, herniation of lung, vascular attenuation present to variable degrees

Differential Diagnosis: Tension pneumothorax

- Location: LUL - 50%
  RML - 24%
  RUL - 18%

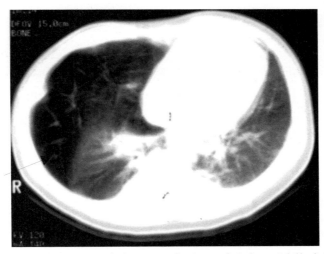

Fig. 32: Axial CT reveals hyperinflation of right middle lobe with passive atelectasis of the lower lobe (arrow)

CONGENITAL CYSTIC ADENOMATOID MALFORMATION (CCAM)

CCAM usually manifests itself in the neonatal period.

10% are manifested in the first year of life.

The basic lesion is a hamartomatous man of fibrous tissue and smooth muscles derived from the terminal respiratory tissues.

Usually involves one lobe. Has normal arterial supply and venous drainage. CCAM constitutes 25% of congenital lung lesion.

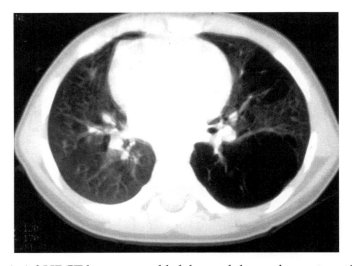

Fig. 33: Axial HRCT lungs reveal left lower lobe coalescent cystic lesion

Radiologic Findings
- Type I—Unilateral, air filled, multicystic lesion
  - Dominant cysts
  - Mass effect
  - Fluid filled, air fluid levels
- Type II—Heterogeneous, uniform small cysts
- Type III—Large and homogeneous
  - Appearance of consolidation

DRUG-INDUCED LUNG DISEASE

Numerous agents including cytotoxic and non-cytotoxic drugs have the potential to affect the lungs adversely. Recognition of drug induced lung disease can be difficult because the clinical manifestation are often non-specific and may be attributed to infection, radiation pneumonitis or recurrence of the underlying disease.

The histopathologic manifestations of drug-induced lung disease are diverse and include patterns of diffuse alveolar damage, bronchiolitis obliterans organizing pneumonia, eosinophilic pneumonia, obliterative bronchiolitis, and pulmonary edema and hemorrhage. Except for a pattern of obliterative bronchiolitis, the remaining four patterns show alveolar filling disorders. Because the clinical and imaging findings of drug-induced lung disease generally reflect the underlying histopathologic process, it is important to be aware of which drugs cause which pattern of histopathology.

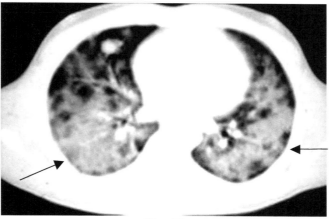

Fig. 34

CT FINDINGS

CT findings show bilateral multifocal alveolar opacity (arrows) resulting from an opioid overdose in a male nurse.

Imaging findings caused by different group of drugs:

Interstitial inflammation	Amiodarone
	Nitrofurantoin
	Methotrexate
	Mexiletine
	Penicillamine
	Tocainide
	Chemotherapy (carmustine [BCNU], mitomycin C, cyclophosphamide, bleomycin, busulfan)
	Beta-lactam, sulfa antibiotics
	Carbamazepine
	Diphenylhydantoin
	NSAIDs

Contd...

Contd...

Noncardiogenic pulmonary edema	Amiodarone Aspirin, NSAID overdose Opiate/hypnotic overdose Tocolytic therapy (terbutaline, isoxsuprine, ritodrine)
Drug-induced SLE	Hydralazine Isoniazid Procainamide Quinidine
Alveolar hemorrhage	Cocaine Penicillamine
Pulmonary infiltrates with eosinophilia	Beta-lactam, sulfa antibiotics Fluoroquinolones

EMPHYSEMA

Areas of low attenuation in the lung caused by permanent abnormal enlargement of air-spaces distal to terminal bronchiole with destruction of their walls. Morphologically classified as centriacinar, panacinar and paraseptal types.

Centrilobular (Centriacinar) Emphysema (CAE)

Multifocal areas of lucency without definite walls, usually surrounding a centrilobular artery. Seen in upper lobes of smokers. Two subtypes are present: (1) Centrilobular emphysema and (2) Focal emphysema. CAE usually involves proximal portion of the acinus in the area of respiratory bronchioles.

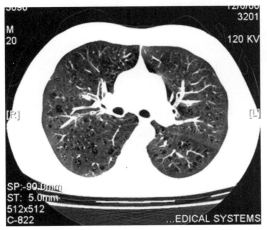

Fig. 35A

Panacinar Emphysema (PAE)

Large areas of lucency with paucity of vascular markings, because of emphysema involving the entire lobule. There is a known association of alpha 1 antitrypsin deficiency and lower lobe PAE.

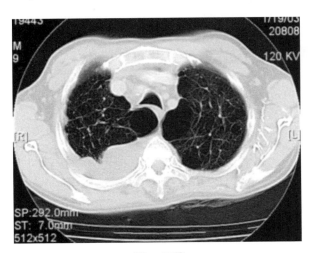

Fig. 35B

Paraseptal Emphysema

Subpleural lucencies due to emphysema involving alveolar ducts and sacs. Common associations—subpleural bullae, spontaneous pneumothorax.

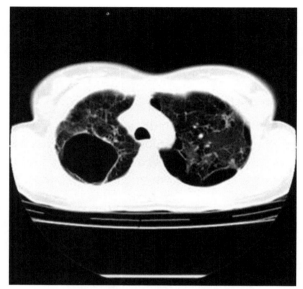

Fig. 35C

Irregular Emphysema

Irregular air space enlargement occurring in patients with TB, sarcoid and fibrotic disease of the lung.

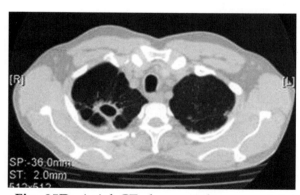

Fig. 35D: Axial CT shows right upper lobe cavity with cicatricial fibrosis causing adjacent emphysematous changes

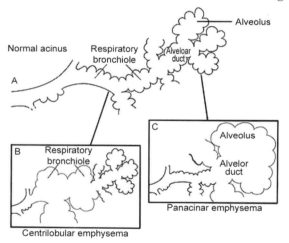

Fig. 35E

CASE 36

EMBOLISM/INFARCTION

Embolus is a clot or mass of foreign material that has been carried by the bloodstream to occlude partly or completely the lumen of a blood vessel. If it occludes the vessel long enough for the tissue distally to die, it produces infarction. Virtually 99% of all emboli represent some part of a dislodged thrombus. Rare forms of emboli include (1) fat embolism, (2) Tumor emboli and (3) Atheromatous—cholesterol emboli.

Unless otherwise proved an embolus should be considered thrombotic in origin. Common cause includes deep vein thrombosis (see Case 91).

Most pulmonary thromboemboli are asymptomatic and produce no detectable changes on a chest radiograph. Roentgenographic findings occur only when a fairly large segmental artery is occluded, when obstruction of many small vessels has impaired pulmonary hemodynamics, or when secondary infarction has occurred.

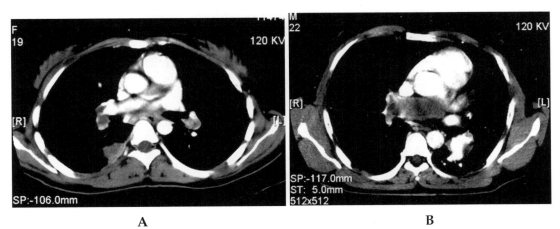

A   B

Figs 36A and B: (A) Axial CECT shows hypodense filling defect in both right and left segmental pulmonary arteries, right midzone peripheral paraspinal pleural based opacity suggestive of an infarct. (B) Axial CECT reveals a large thrombus filling the right main pulmonary artery

CT FINDINGS

CT findings are that of a luminal filling defect within the main or segmental pulmonary artery. Parenchymal changes include increased and decreased lung attenuation as well as wedge shaped pleural based areas of parenchymal consolidation, linear bands and atelectasis, pleural effusion.

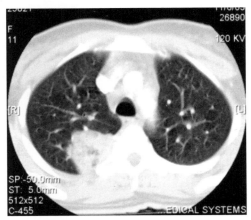

Fig. 36C: Axial CT reveals a wedge shaped peripheral opacity in the right upperlobe posterior segment suggestive of a infarct

CASE 37

ENDOBRONCHIAL OBSTRUCTION

Endobronchial obstruction results in resorption atelectasis, they cause a spectrum of abnormalities reflecting the nature of the primary abnormalities. They can cause retention of secretions with increased density. And become wedge shaped. Chronic obstruction can cause cicatricial changes.

Endobronchial obstruction can be classified as:

1. Neoplasm—Bronchogenic carcinoma, bronchial carcinoid, adenoid cystic carcinoma.
2. Metastasis—kidney, breast, colon, lymphoma.
3. Non-neoplastic lesions include—Mucus plug, foreign body, TB/fungal lesions.
4. Extrinsic lesion—Enlarged lymph nodes due to TB, sarcoidosis.

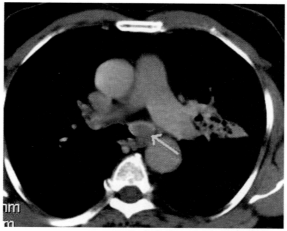

Fig. 37A: Axial CECT section at carinal level shows a hypodense, non-enhancing, oval soft tissue lesion impacted in the left main bronchus with distal obstructive changes in the lingula. In this case it was extracted via bronchoscopy and found to be arecanut

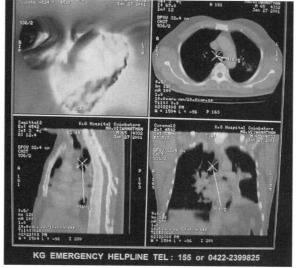

Fig. 37B: Virtual bronchoscopy images showing the impacted foreign body in the left main bronchus (same patient as in Fig. 37A)

END-STAGE LUNG

End-stage lung—final stage in progression of lung disease with honeycombing, extensive cystic changes, conglomerate fibrosis and disruption of normal lung architecture. In this part of the world, most cases result from a progressive primary infection or from inadequately treated prolonged post primary TB. Severe fibrosis with volume loss, hilar retraction and secondary tracheomegaly. Bronchiectasis is often noted.

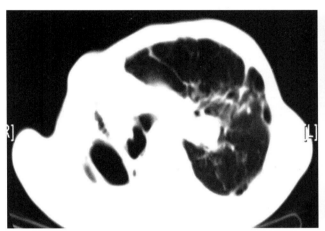 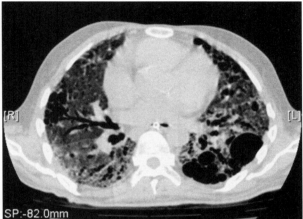

Figs 38A and B: (A) Axial CT shows end stage cavitary changes of the right lung with hyperinflation of left lung showing fibrotic changes. (B) Axial CT shows multiple cysts suggestive of honeycombing with areas of fibrosis and alveolitis

CT FINDINGS

CT findings depend on the nature of the primary disease—in case of TB or chronic inflammatory disease extensive fibrosis with cicatricial ectasia is noted (Fig. 38A).

In case of immunological diseases a predominant *Honeycombing* with a fibrotic pattern is seen (Fig. 38B). Relatively preserved lung shows hyperinflatory changes.

CASE 39

EWING'S TUMOR

Most common malignant tumor of the bone in children. Peak incidence is around 15 years of age.

Presentation

- Severe localized pain
- Soft tissue mass
- Fever, leukocytosis, anemia.

Location

Ribs (6%), Humerus (10%), Femur (25%).

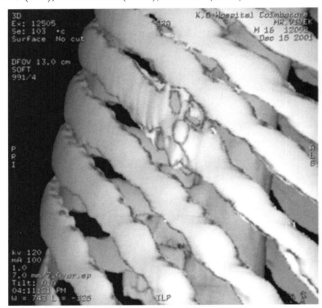 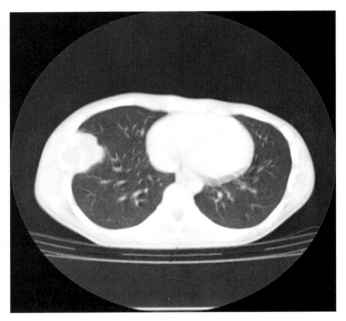

Figs 39A and B: (A) SSD of ribs showing an expansile osteolytic lesion of the 8th rib. (B) Axial CT showing soft tissue component of the rib lesion (biopsy suggestive of a Ewing's sarcoma)

CT FINDINGS

CT appearance is that of a focal osteolytic lesion of rib with soft tissue component (arrow).

Differential Diagnosis

1. Osteomyelitis
2. Eosinophilic granuloma
3. Spindle cell sarcoma
4. Metastatic carcinoma.

CASE 40

FUNGAL ABSCESS

Fungi are relatively uncommon causes of pneumonia but are of increasing importance as the prevalence of immunocompromised patients increase. The pathogens causing fungal pneumonias can be divided into two groups, those that require an immunocompromised host to cause disease and those that can cause disease in normal hosts but lead to more severe disease in immunocompromised patients. The pathogens associated with immunodeficient patients are *Aspergillus* spp., *Candida* spp., *Cryptococcus neoformans*, and the zygomycetes. The other agents associated with fungal pneumonias are the so-called endemic mycoses — *Coccidioides immitis*, *Histoplasma capsulatum* and *Blastomyces dermatitidis*. Aspergillus infection is the most common pulmonary fungal disease. Common finding in tissue invasive fungal disease are thickwalled irregular cavity with areas of consolidation with or without pleural effusion.

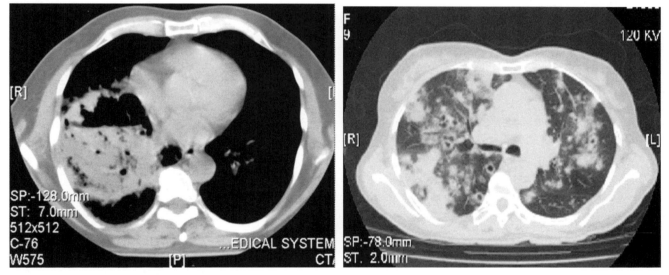

Figs 40A and B: (A) Axial CT shows a left midzone cavitary lesion with irregular margins with air fluid level in apatient with uncontrolled diabetic—mucormycosis. (B) Axial CT in a immunocompromised patient showing multiple cavitary nodules with associated alveolar opacities—proved to be a case of invasive aspergillosis

CASE 41

FISSURAL FLUID

Fissural loculation of fluid give rise to pseudotumors, usually seen in patients with congestive cardiac failure. Loculation implies adherence of pleural layers in peripheral portion of fissure, secondary to previous inflammatory disease.

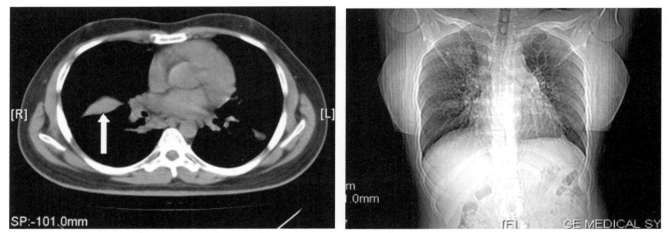

Figs 41A and B

CT FINDINGS

CT demonstrates fluid within the fissures, appearance varies with the quantity, spindle shaped if limited to the fissure and triangular if in communication with the pleural cavity.

GROUND GLASS OPACITY

Hazy increase in lung opacity without obscuration of underlying vessels. Represents active or acute disease and is due to minimal interstitial thickening or air space filling or both.

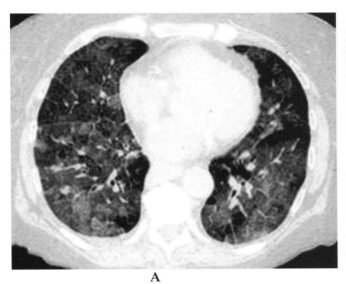 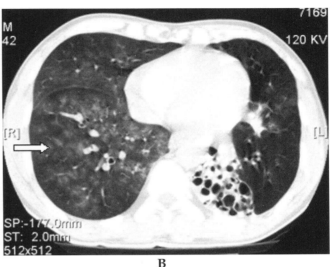

A   B

Figs 42A and B: (A) Axial CT lung shows bilateral diffuse ground glass attenuation in the lower lobe in a patient with desquamative alveolitis. (B) Axial CT shows right lower lobe multifocal patchy alveolar opacity (arrow) due to hemorrhage in a patient with left lower lobe bronchiectasis

Causes of a Diffuse Pattern of GGO on CT Scanning	Causes of a Focal Pattern of GGO on CT Scanning (Fig. 42A)
• Acute rejection of lung transplantation • Adult respiratory distress syndrome • Edema • Extrinsic allergic alveolitis • Hemorrhage • Infectious pneumonia	• Bronchiolitis obliterans organizing pneumonia (BOOP) • Bronchoalveolar lavage • Bronchoalveolar cell carcinoma • Hemorrhage • Pulmonary infection

CASE 43

HONEYCOMBING

Cystic spaces with sizes ranging from few mm to few cm with well-defined fibrous shared walls. Usually subpleural and forming several layers. Associated with pulmonary fibrosis. Hall mark finding in fibrosing parenchymal lung disease.

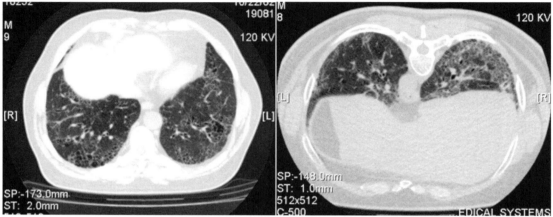

Figs 43A and B: Axial supine and prone HRCT of the lungs reveals bilateral subpleural conglomerate cysts suggestive of honeycombing

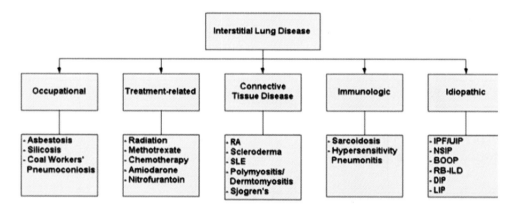

COMMON CONDITIONS PRESENTING WITH HONEYCOMBING AND RETICULATION

CT FINDINGS WITH ASSOCIATED PATHOLOGY

Small cystic spaces with thick walls that begin subpleurally (see left lung)	Irregular thickening of bronchovascular bundles in regions of fibrosis
Air bronchiolograms (traction bronchiolectasis) embedded in areas of increased attenuation	Traction bronchiectasis and bronchiolectasis
Irregular, reticular appearing increased subpleural attenuation (both lungs)	Minor component of ground glass attenuation, usually associated with regions of fibrosis

HYPERSENSITIVE PNEUMONITIS

Hypersensitivity pneumonitis (HP), also known as extrinsic allergic alveolitis, is characterized by chronic granulomatous inflammation in response to repeated inhalation of environmental antigens. HP has been associated with a wide range of antigens including mammalian and avian proteins, various bacteria, fungi and drugs like nitrofurantoin, sulfonamides, erythromycin.

Radiographic abnormalities listed below generally are distributed in the mid-toupper lung zones.

Acute and Subacute

- Can be normal in acute disease
- Diffuse increased parenchymal density (ground glass attenuation)
- Mosaic attenuation (best seen on expiratory scans; represents air-trapping)
- Patchy or diffuse air space consolidation
- Diffuse, ill-defined nodules often < 5 mm

Chronic (findings can mimic idiopathic pulmonary fibrosis)

- Ground-glass opacities
- Mosaic attenuation with evidence of air-trapping
- Diffuse reticular opacities
- Parenchymal micronodules
- Loss of lung volume
- Honeycombing-emphysema

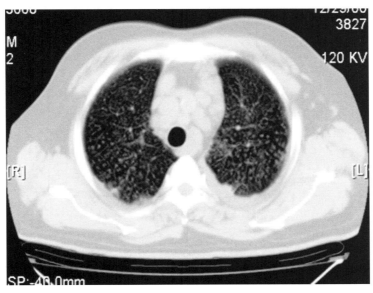

Fig. 44A: Subacute: Axial CT lungs shows bilateral multiple mid size nodular opacity in a patient working in a textile mill

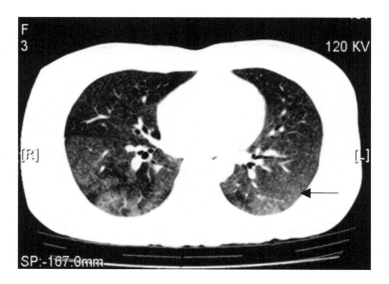

Fig. 44B: Acute: Axial CT lung shows bilateral midzone air space (arrow) consolidation in a patient with atopy

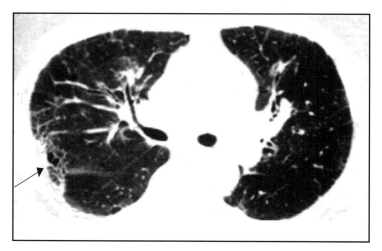

Fig. 44C: Chronic: Axial CT shows right upperzone peripheral honeycombing with adjacent early fibrotic changes (arrow)

CASE 45

PULMONARY HEMORRHAGE

Diffuse pulmonary hemorrhage is characterized by widespread parenchymal hemorrhage from the microvasculature of the lung and occurs in a large group of disorders. The disorders have overlapping features of glomerulonephritis, immune complex, and antiglomerular basement membrane disease.

Acute pulmonary hemorrhage appears as areas of ground glass opacity or sometimes as frank consolidation on **HRCT.** These abnormalities usually resolve rapidly during remission. Discrete pulmonary nodules of uniform size are identifiable in patients whose CT scans are obtained during complete or partial clinical remission. Focal accumulation of hemosiderin and hemosiderin-laden macrophages within alveoli may give a nodular appearance on **HRCT.**

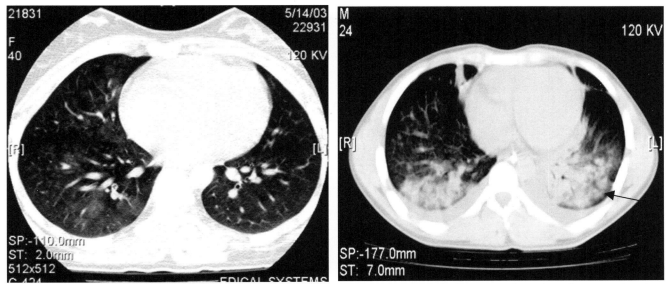

Figs 45A and B: (A) Axial CT in lung window shows bilateral lower lobe patchy alveolar opacity in a patient with hemoptysis (case of Goodpasture's syndrome). (B) Axial CT shows bilateral lower lobe alveolar opacity (arrow) in a patient with leptospirosis patient presented with hemoptysis

Differential Diagnosis
- Infectious pneumonia
- Pulmonary edema
- Pulmonary hemorrhage
- Acute or subacute hypersensitivity pneumonitis
- Desquamative interstitial pneumonitis
- Pulmonary alveolar proteinosis

Causes of Hemoptysis	
Infectious	Bronchitis, bronchiectasis, TB, lung abscess, mycetoma
Neoplasms	Foreign bodies/Trauma
Cardiovascular	Mitral stenosis, Pulmonary embolus, LV failure
Other	AVM's, vasculitis, idiopathic hemosiderosis, catamenial, Goodpasture's

CAUSES OF INTRAALVEOLAR HEMORRHAGE
Idiopathic pulmonary hemosiderosis Goodpasture's syndrome Blood dyscrasias with thrombocytopenia Anticoagulants Disseminated intravascular coagulation Pulmonary contusion from blunt trauma

HYPERLUCENT HEMITHORAX

This condition results from a insult to the developing lung, small bronchi are affected in addition to bronchioles, the abnormal lung remains inflated by collateral air drift, and giving rise to the key finding of unilateral or segmental lucency.

Diffuse air trapping can be easily overlooked because the lungs are uniformly involved. Attenuation of lung is lower than normal often with values in the -900 H range rather than –600 to –750 Hounsfield unit. These changes are subtle and can be overlooked unless measured.

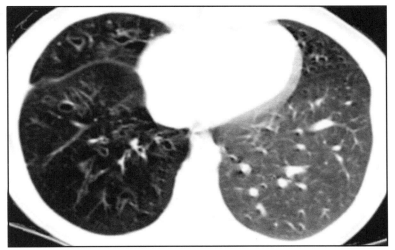

Fig. 46

SWYER-JAMES SYNDROME results from bronchiolitis obliterans secondary to an infectious insult to the small airways, typically occurring before 8 years of age, before alveolar development is complete. It should be emphasized that postinfectious bronchiolitis obliterans can occur at any age; this particular syndrome refers to that which occurs in childhood. It was first described as a radiographic entity by Swyer and James in 1953. The classic constellation of radiographic findings include hyperlucent lung, small ipsilateral hilum with decreased peripheral pulmonary vascularity, and air trapping. Adenovirus has been implicated as the primary agent. A wide variety of other organisms have been described, however, including measles, *Mycobacterium tuberculosis*, pertussis, and *Mycoplasma pneumonia*. Although the diagnosis can often be made by classic findings on inspiratory-expiratory chest radiographs, patients presenting with atypical radiographic or clinical findings can create a more difficult diagnostic dilemma.

In the pediatric age group, CT scanning can help differentiate between several diagnostic possibilities including endobronchial foreign bodies, extrinsic compression of a bronchus by a congenital cyst or neoplasm, pulmonary agenesis or hypoplasia, compensatory emphysema, or congenital lobar emphysema.

Expiratory **HRCT** (Fig. 46) scanning in patients with Swyer-James syndrome can show multifocal bilateral air trapping that is not seen or is underappreciated on conventional radiographs or CT scans. Patients may be entirely asymptomatic with this syndrome, but may also suffer from recurrent respiratory infections and hemoptysis.

CASE 47

LYMPHANGIOLEIOMYOMATOSIS

An uncommon condition characterised by the following clinical presentation:

• Occurs exclusively in women of reproductive years
• Presents with progressive dyspnea, chylous pleural effusion, hemoptysis, massive hemorrhage and recurrent pneumothorax.

Pathology

Disorderly proliferation of smooth muscle, bronchioles, alveolar septa, arteries, veins and lymphatics.

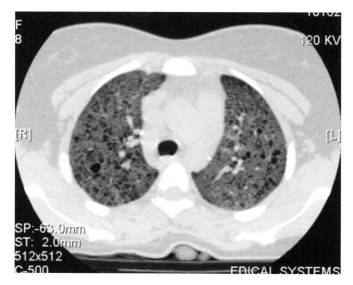

Fig. 47: Axial HRCT lungs reveal bilateral diffuse discrete thin walled cysts

CT FINDINGS

• Numerous thin-walled cysts, intervening lung normal
• Diffuse, bilateral involvement
• Adenopathy
• Pleural effusion
• Increase in lung volume.

Differential Diagnosis

Tuberous sclerosis, Langerhan's pulmonary histiocytosis and emphysema.

CASE 48

LYMPHANGITIC CARCINOMATOSIS

It is a common form of spread of carcinoma within the lung, both primary and metastatic. The term implies the presence of tumor in sites associated with lymphatic vessels, i.e. the interstitial tissue surrounding bronchi, bronchioles and pulmonary arteries, and within the bronchial mucosa, the interlobular septa and the pleura. In the case of primary pulmonary carcinoma or metastatic carcinoma involving hilar/bronchopulmonary lymph nodes, the carcinoma extends directly into the adjacent lymphatics/interstitial tissue. In the case of metastatic carcinoma that reaches the lung via the pulmonary arterial circulation, tumor cells within minute emboli cross the vessel wall into the perivascular interstitium.

Among primary pulmonary carcinomas, lymphangitic carcinomatosis is most commonly seen in adenocarcinoma and small cell carcinoma. Often it is focal and localized to the interstitial tissue within 1 to 2 cm of the tumor or, in the case of small cell carcinoma, is associated with obstructive pneumonitis; thus, radiologic findings related to the spread are often not apparent. Although the pattern of spread may be seen with virtually any metastatic carcinoma, it is most frequently associated with breast, stomach, and prostate primaries.

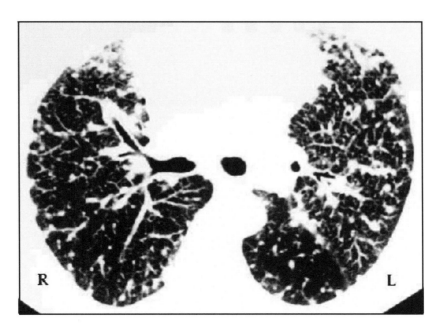

Fig. 48: Metastasis due to carcinoma stomach

CT FINDINGS

Bilateral nodular septal thickening (patient with carcinoma stomach presented to us with dyspnea).

Most commonly bilateral and diffuse involvement of the lungs.

Characteristic abnormalities consist of thickening of interlobular septa and thickening of peribronchovascular and subpleural interstitium.There is preservation of normal lung architecture. The thickened septa may be smooth or usually have beaded or nodular appearance due to tumor growth along the lymphatics. Discrete small nodules may also be present. Pleural effusion and lymphadenopathy may also be present.

MILIARY PATTERN

A condition of the lung characterized by Miliary nodules is a well-known chest radiograph pattern, consistent with the presence of multiple nodules in the lung.

A heterogeneous group of conditions comprising more than 80 entities may display this pattern.

These characteristic nodules are small, usually 1 to 3 mm in diameter, and have sharp margins.

Three types of distribution have been described: centrilobular, perilymphatic, and random.

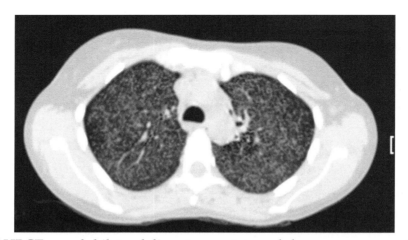

Fig. 49: Axial HRCT reveals bilateral discrete punctate nodules—proven case of miliary TB

Differential Diagnosis and Algorithm

See the pullout.

MOSAIC PERFUSION

Inhomogenous attenuation of lung parenchyma with focal regions of lucency which show smaller size of vessels. May be due to vascular obstruction, abnormal ventilation or airways disease.

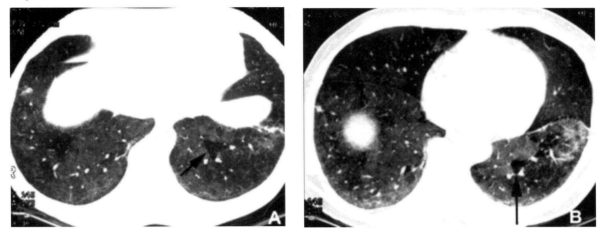

Figs 50A and B

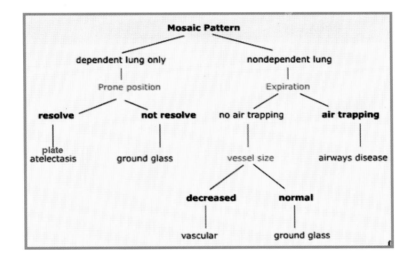

CT FINDINGS

End-expiratory images help to determine whether mosaic perfusion is caused by air-trapping or primary vascular disease.

Airway disease		Primary vascular disease	
Inspiratory image	**Expiratory image**	**Inspiratory image**	**Expiratory image**
Light lung	becomes lighter	Light lung	becomes lighter
Dark lung	stays dark	Dark lung	becomes lighter

MIDDLE LOBE SYNDROME

Definition: Chronic collapse of middle lobe or lingular lobe, mostly occurring as a post inflammatory sequelae. Predisposing factors for collapse of middle lobe and lingula include:

a. Presence of many lymph nodes surrounding their stem bronchi

b. Reduced collateral drift to the middle lobe in those with complete major and minor fissures.

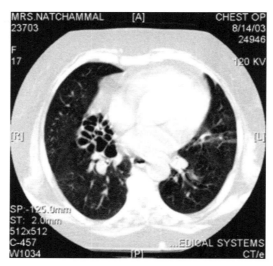

Fig. 51: Axial HRCT lung reveals cystic bronchiectatic changes involving the medial segment of right middle lobe

Etiology of Middle Lobe Syndrome

Chronic inflammatory disease probably prior pneumonia with poor clearance due to poor collateral air drift. Previously thought to be due to compression by tuberculous lymph node.

Complication: Long standing atelectasis leading to bronchiectasis.

CT FINDINGS

Atelectasis manifested as triangular opacity abutting the cardiac border with volume loss, with or without bronchiectatic changes.

MESOTHELIOMA

Uncommon neoplasm accounting less than 5% of pleural malignancies. There is association between asbestosis (crocidolite) and mesothelioma. Other causes include chronic inflammation (TB, empyema), irradiation. Peak age incidence is around 50-70 years.

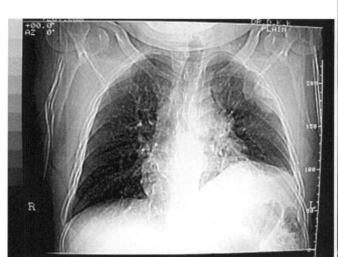 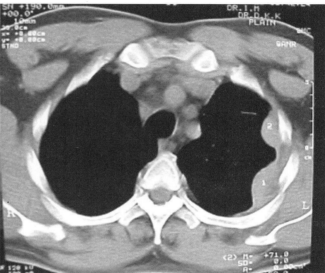

Fig. 52

Pathophysiology

Characteristically mesothelioma permeates the pleural space, causing pleura to become markedly thickened, irregular and nodular. The tumor often encircles the lung causing entrapment. Effusions are often present.

   Mesotheliomas may rarely present as more localized masses mimicking a benign fibrous tumor. Diagnosis is by histopathology as there is no CT specific signs for mesothelioma as any malignancy involving the pleura can simulate these appearances.

CT FINDINGS

Pleural thickening, pleural effusion with ipsilateral mediastinal shift, calcified pleural plaques.

Differential Diagnosis

Pleural fibrosis from infection (TB, fungal, actinomycosis), fibrothorax, empyema, metastatic adenocarcinoma.

NEOPLASIA

A benign or malignant tumor of the lung or its contents. The usual culprits are bronchogenic carcinoma or pulmonary metastases from some other primary tumor.

The classic finding is a mass. This may be hard to see if the lesion is small or if it is obscured by other processes accompanying the tumor, such as pleural effusion or atelectasis. CT is very helpful in the workup of suspected lung tumor.

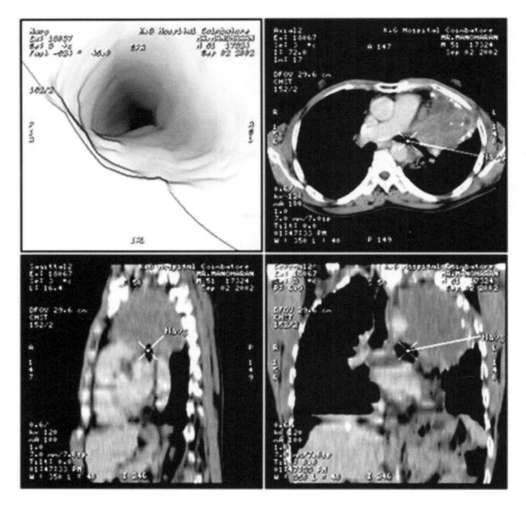

Fig. 53

BRONCHOGENIC CARCINOMA

Clinical Presentation —10% asymptomatic, cough, pneumonia.

Paraneoplastic syndrome—Cachexia, clubbing, inappropriate ADH secretion.

Thrombophlebitis, non-bacterial thrombotic endocarditis.

Staging

Ti	Ca in situ, rare
T1	<3 cm, none near main bronchus or pleura
T2	Abuting visceral pleura, greater than 2 cm from carina, causing atel or >3 cm
T3	Out of lung, within 2 cm of carina without involving the carina
	No vital structure invaded, resec poss
T4	Vital structure invaded, no resection
	Vital includes esoph, carina, trachea, heart, vert body
Tx	Malig eff or sputum, stage IV automatically
N1	intrapulmonary nodes
N2	Mediastinal, ipsilateral only
N3	Any nodes in vicinity inc supraclavicular or scalene
M1	Any dist mets, only 1/3 of adrenal abn actually mets
Stage 1	T2 N0 M0
Stage 2	T2 N1 M0
Stage 3a	T3 N2 M0, last chance for resection
Stage 3b	T4 N3 M0, nonresectable
Stage 4	M1 or Tx

1. **Adenocarcinoma**—50%, arise in bronchiolar or alveolar epithelium
   Mucin or psammoma bodies seen on histology
   Destroys tissue as it grows, may be endobronchial
   Slow to grow but shows early metastasis. Shows a irregular and spiculated appearance, with surrounding fibrosis. Borders can have any appearance, do not define malignancy known to arise from previous scars, rarely cavitates.

   Bronchioalveolar—A well differentiated type of adenocarcinoma with pneumonic pattern spreads on existing bronchiole and alveolar walls without disruption
   90% form single isolated nodule of ill defined density which can fragment and redistribute forming multi-focal infiltrates, may simulate Pneumonia or a diffuse nodular pattern
   Good prognosis if resected as a solitary pattern.

2. **Squamous Cell Ca** - 35%, arises centrally in lobar or segmental bronchi
   Rapid growth but metastasis late, good prognosis
   Lesion is polypoidal and grow into the wall and lumen causing cough and hemoptysis
   Central necrosis frequent, cavitates if communication to the bronchus is established.

3. **Small Cell Ca**—25%, arise centrally in main or lobar bronchi, thought to arise from Kulchitsky cells, early peribronchial invasion causing extrinsic compression and obstruction. Lymphatics invaded early, enlarged nodes lead to hematogenous spread.
   SVC obstruction a frequent feature. Strong association with smoking.

4. **Large Cell Ca**—15%, Dx of exclusion, usually peripheral and large at time of diagnosis > 3 cm
   Poorly differentiated, rapid growth, early metastasis, poor prognosis, frequently shows central necrosis.

5. **Pancoast's Tumor**—Squamous or adenocarcinoma arising in superior sulcus, diagnosis is by symptom—invasion into brachial plexus and sympathetic ganglion chain. Causing arm pain and Horner's syndrome. CXR—apical fibrous cap >5 mm and rib destruction.

RARE PRIMARY NEOPLASMS OF THE LUNG

Bronchial Adenomas - True bronchial gland adenomas or rare.
Carcinoid accounts for 90% of adenomas, most are central and present with hemoptysis, 90% are < 50 yrs.
CT Very marginated, may also be endobronchial, calcification in 30%, present as recurrent pneumonia, etc. 15% met to local nodes.

Adenoid Cystic Carcinoma—Commonly in trachea
Slow growing, sharply marginated
Often locally invasive due to lack of symptom.

Mucoepidermoid Carcinoma—Variable aggressive
Abundant mucinous cysts and solid collections of squamous cells
Slow growing, can be exophytic
Carcinosarcoma—Aggressive with local invasion and early metastasis
Epithelial and mesenchymal components seen in same tumor. Presents as peripheral lung mass with necrosis and hemorrhage.
Central endobronchial type may simulate mucous plug.

CASE 54

NODULES

A focal rounded opacity of varying sizes may have well or ill-defined margins.
See the flow sheets in the appendix for approach to nodules.

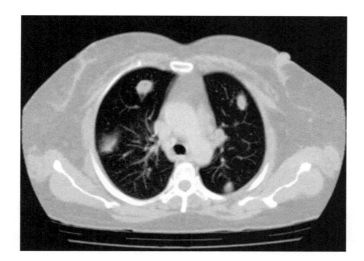

Fig. 54A: Axial CT showing multiple large nodules
(diabetic patient with *Staph. pneumoniae*)

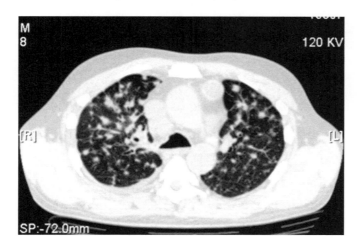

Fig. 54B: Axial CT lung shows multiple well marginated nodules in a
perlymphatic distribution (case of Ca colon with metastasis)

CASE 55

OBSTRUCTIVE HYPERINFLATION

Obstructive hyperinflation characterized by increase in lung volume.

Caused by partial bronchial obstruction due to:

    Aspirated foreign body

    Bronchial stenosis

    Bronchomalacia

    Broncholith

    Adjacent lymph node

Mechanism—Air trapping due to ball valve obstruction. Diagnosis is usually evident on expiratory CT—where there is persistence of decreased lung attenuation.

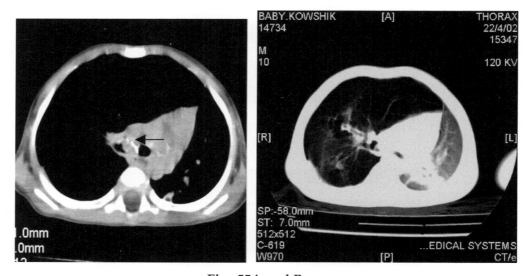

Figs 55A and B

CT FINDINGS

Persistence of decreased attenuation of the entire right lung in expiratory phase due to air trapping secondary to compression of right main bronchus by calcified retrocarinal lymph node (Fig. 55A, arrow).

CASE 56

PARENCHYMAL BAND-LINEAR

Peripheral opacity, 2-5 cm in length making contact with the pleural surface. Seen in patients with lung fibrosis, most commonly asbestosis and sarcoidosis.

These parenchymal bands represent one of the following:
a. Areas of peribronchovascular fibrosis
b. Atelectasis associated with lung or pleural fibrosis

Parenchymal bands are seen in
a. Asbestosis
b. Sarcoidosis with interstitial fibrosis
c. Silicosis
d. CWP
e. Tuberculosis

Differential Diagnosis

Diagnosis	Features of parenchymal bands
Asbestosis	Multiple parenchymal bands with pleural and septal thickening, basal
Sarcoidosis	Parenchymal bands associated with septal thickening
Silicosis and CWP	Associated PMF and emphysema seen
Tuberculosis	Associated with scarring

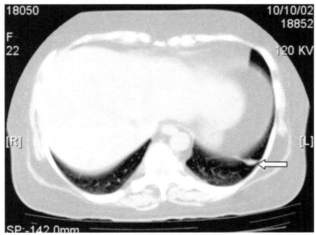
Fig. 56

HRCT findings—Long bands, several mm thick, irregular in contour, making contact with the pleura and associated with distorted lung parenchyma and bronchovascular structures.

CASE 57

PANCOAST TUMOR

Definition: Superior pulmonary sulcus tumor.

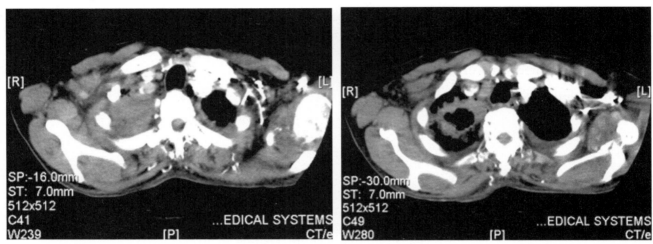

Figs 57A and B: Right upper lobe apical soft tissue density lesion with cavitary changes

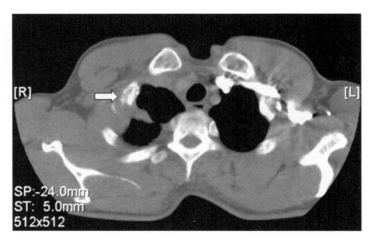

Fig. 57C: Osteolytic lesion in the right first rib with adjacent
soft tissue lesion (arrow)

- Constitutes around 3% of primary lung tumors
  - Usually squamous cell carcinoma
  - Pancoast syndrome—caused by superior sulcus tumor invading lower cords of brachial plexus and sympathetic stellate ganglion
  - Consists of clinical triad of
    a. ipsilateral arm pain
    b. wasting of hand muscles
    c. Horner's syndrome

- There is usually associated local destruction of bone
- They can involve
  a. Adjacent chest wall
  b. Brachial plexus
  c. Subclavian vessels
  d. Spine
- Presents as apical pleural thickening with or without destruction of adjacent ribs and spine or as a discrete intrapulmonary mass in the lung apex with pleural and bone involvement. Cavitation may be present.

CASE 58

PLEURAL CALCIFICATION

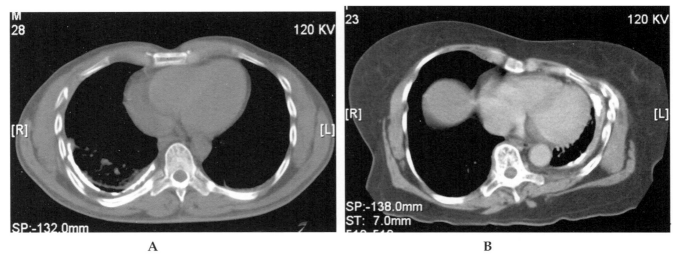

A   B

Fig. 58

CT FINDINGS

Plain CT shows sheet of pleural thickening in the right (Fig. 58A) and left (Fig. 58B) basal pleura. Prominent extra pleural fat pad is reflective of a chronic inflammatory sequelae. Both patients had past history of treatment for tuberculosis.

Causes

   i. Tuberculosis
  ii. Empyema
 iii. Hemothorax
 iv. Asbestosis
  v. Talc
 vi. Scleroderma

Calcifications along the diaphragmatic pleura which are bilateral but asymmetric are pathognomonic of asbestosis, associated pleural plaques.

PLEURAL THICKENING

Defined as smooth un interrupted pleural density extending over atleast one-fourth of the chest wall, with or without obliteration of the cardiophrenic angle.

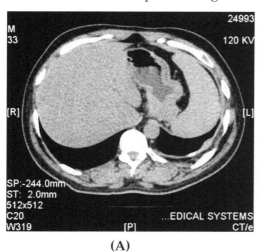 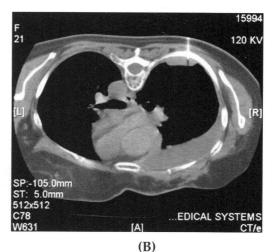

(A)   (B)

Figs 59A and B: (A) Plain CT shows diffuse thickening of parietal pleural in a patient with a history of treatment for empyema. (B) Plain CT in prone for biopsy of a focal pleural deposit (biopsy was suggestive of metastatic adenocarcinoma)

CT FINDINGS

On CT diffuse pleural thickening is defined as continuous sheet of pleural thickening more than 5 cm wide, 8 cm in craniocaudal extent and more than 3 mm thick.

Causes

1. Fibrothorax—usually almost 2 cm in thickness, due to formation of dense fibrous layer on the visceral pleura which may calcify. Seen in
   a. Organizing effusion
   b. Hemothorax
   c. Pyothorax
2. Infection
   a. Chronic empyema- over bases
   b. Tuberculosis- over lung apex with apical cavity
   c. Histoplasmosis
   d. Aspergilloma
3. Collagen vascular disease, e.g. rheumatoid arthritis
4. Pneumoconiosis
   a. Asbestosis
   b. Talcosis
5. Neoplasm
   a. Metastases
   b. Diffuse malignant mesothelioma
   c. Pancoast tumor
   d. Focal mesenchymal tumor
6. Rare cause—Pleural hyaloserositis

PLEURAL EFFUSION

A state characterized by the presence of fluid within the pleural space. Many things can cause this, and there may or may not be additional findings on the chest film that will steer one toward the cause.

Blunting of the costophrenic angles on the PA film or of the posterior costophrenic sulci on the lateral film, widening of a fissure, and layering along the chest wall.

Decubitus views can be very useful for demonstrating mobility of an effusion. In my opinion, bilateral decubitus views should always be ordered so that one can not only assess the presence and mobility of an effusion, but also demonstrate lesions of the lung parenchyma hidden by the effusion.

CT can demonstrate small effusions and identify pulmonary or other pleural disease masked by larger effusions. This is especially helpful if plain radiographs are difficult to interpret.

Thoracentesis for cultures and chemistries may be helpful.

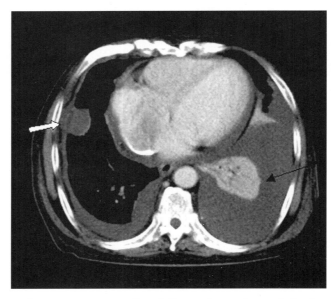

Fig. 60: CECT in a patient with congestive cardiac failure shows large left pleural effusion in the left side with passive atelectasis of lung (black arrow). Right side fissural fluid is present (white arrow)

PNEUMATOCELE

Definition: Thin walled welldefined lucency within the lung, associated with acute pneumonia, invariably transient.

- Does not indicate destruction of lung parenchyma
- Transient, occurs during healing phase
- Spontaneous resolution is the norm
- Usually multiple
- Commonest complication- pneumothorax
- May get infected- air fluid levels

Pathogenesis

a. Severe distension of small bronchioles
b. Evacuated focus of necrotic lung
c. Air from ruptured alveoli dissect along interstitium to form subpleural air cyst

Causes

a. Infective
   a. Staphylococcus
   b. *Pneumocystis carinii*
   c. Klebsiella
   d. *E. coli*
   e. Pneumococcus
b. Non-infective
   a. Traumatic
   b. Hydrocarbon ingestion

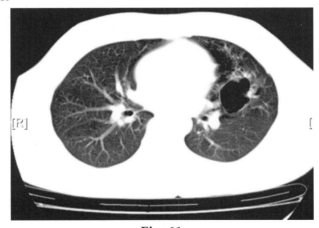

Fig. 61

CT FINDINGS

Axial CT shows a well-defined cystic space in the left lingua (follow-up case of pneumoniae).

PNEUMOTHORAX

A state characterized by the presence of gas within the pleural space.

The only direct sign is identification of a visceral pleural line. An air-fluid level in the hemithorax provides indirect evidence of a hydropneumothorax.

Classification

- Traumatic
- Iatrogenic
  - Thoracotomy
  - Percutaneous biopsy
  - Mechanical ventilation
- Spontaneous
  - Primary (70%)—normal appearing lung
  - Secondary—underlying lung disease

Secondary Spontaneous Pneumothorax

Etiology
- Bullous emphysema
- Infiltrative lung disease
- Eosinophilic granuloma
- Lymphangioleiomyomatosis
- Infectious diseases
- Malignant neoplasia

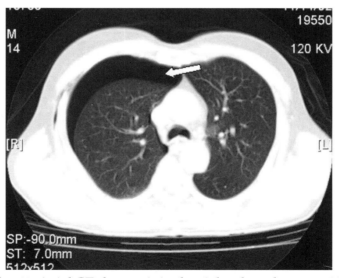

Fig. 62: Axial CT shows air in the right pleural space with passive collapse of the lung (arrow)

Primary Spontaneous Pneumothorax

- 0.3 to 0.8% of hospital admissions
- Male : Female 3:1
- Ages 20 to 40
- Tall, thin individuals
- ? Rupture of small apical blebs
- Recurrence: 20%

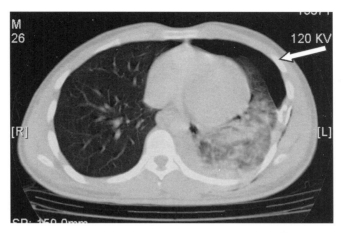

Fig. 62.B: Axial CT reveals left lowerlobe patchy alveolar opacity suggestive of parenchymal contusion with pneumothorax (arrow). Patient had sustained a road traffic accident the previous day.

PLEURAL DEPOSITS

Diffuse or focal pleural thickening with lobulated borders

- May be solitary or multiple
- May be unilateral or bilateral
- Usually accompanied by pleural effusion

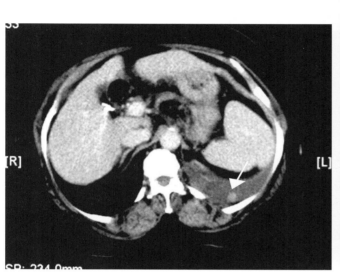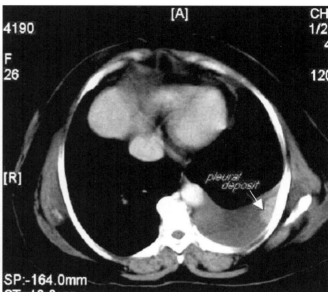

Figs 63A and B: Axial CT chest in mediastinal window shows left pleural effusion with enhancing pleural nodules (arrows)—case of carcinoma breast with pleural metastasis

Causes

a. Loculated pleural collection (infectious/hemorrhagic)
b. Malignant mesothelioma
c. Metastases
- Lung-40%
- Breast-20%
- Invasive thymoma

CASE 64

PULMONARY CONTUSION

The exudation of edema fluid and blood into the parenchyma of the lung in both its air-space and interstitial components, and is the most common pulmonary complication of blunt chest trauma.

CT appearance varies from patchy, irregular areas of opacity to diffuse and extensive homogeneous consolidation. Onset is almost invariably within 6 hours of trauma, and usually resolves within 3 or 4 days.

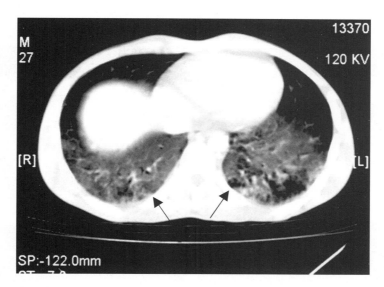

Fig. 64: Axial CT lungs in a case of Road traffic accident reveals bilateral
lower lobes alveolar opacities

Results from direct transmission of energy through the chest wall to the underlying lung resulting in injury to alveoli and interstitium. Appears as unilateral or bilateral patchy airspace disease which tends to be peripheral, non-segmental and geographic in distribution.

PULMONARY EDEMA

Exudation of fluid from the capillaries into the interstitial tissues and air spaces of the lungs. This process is multifactorial.

Radiographic findings depend on whether the edema fluid remains relatively localized in the interstitial spaces or whether it also occupies the air spaces of the lung as well. If interstitial, one may see thickening of the interlobular septa (Kerley lines). If it occupies the air spaces, findings range from patchy ill-defined opacities to more confluent opacity.

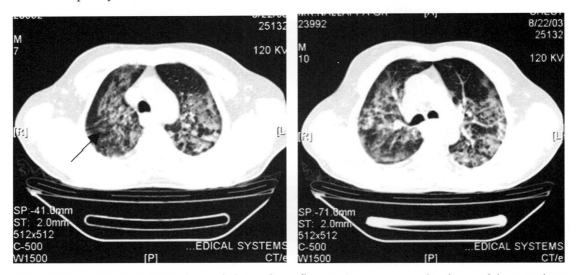

Figs 65A and B: Axial CT shows bilateral confluent air space opacity (arrow) in a patient with renal failure and clinical features of pulmonary edema

Radiological Pattern for Pulmonary Edema

Radiological sign	Cardiogenic	Renal	Capillary injury
Heart shape	L-sided enlargement	R and L enlargement	Normal
Vascular pedicle width (SV)	+	++	Normal
Pulmonary blood distribution	Balanced or inverted	Balanced	Normal
Pulmonary blood volume	Normal or +	++	Normal
Septal lines	++	+	No
Peribronchial and vessel cuffing	+	+	No
Air bronchogram	+	+	++
Lung opacity distribution	Central and peripheral	Central	Peripheral and central
Pleural effusion	++	+	Uncommon
Soft-tissue chest wall	+	++	Normal

CASE 66

PNEUMOCYSTIS CARINII PNEUMONIA

Pneumocystis carinii pneumonia is a significant cause of HIV associated pneumoniae.
Seen in patients with cd4 count less than 200 cells/cu mm.

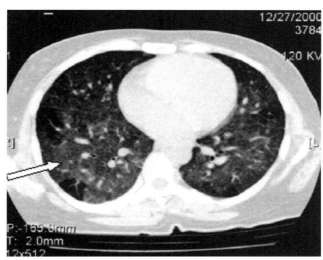

Fig. 66

HRCT FINDINGS

The major manifestation of PCP on HRCT is diffuse, bilateral, ground-glass opacity. In the early phase of infection, minimal reticulation may be present. As the disease progresses, linear opacity and reticulation, due to interlobular septal thickening, become increasingly prominent. In patients with severe disease, diffuse air-space consolidation is often encountered. *Pneumatoceles* are often encountered on HRCT studies in patients with PCP.

Pulmonary Conditions and Infections Associated with AIDS		
Common	*Less common*	*Occasionally seen*
Bacterial pneumonia	*M.avium* complex	Toxoplasmosis
Pneumocystis carinii pneumonia	Cryptococcosis	Cryptosporism
Mycobacterium tuberculosis	Coccidioidomycosis	Strongyloides
Kaposi's sarcoma	Histoplasmosis	*M. kansasii*
	Cytomegalovirus	Legionella
	Nocardia	Aspergillus
	Lymphoma	Lymphoid and nonspecific interstitial pneumonitis

PULMONARY LACERATION

Common chest injury caused by

a. Shearing injury caused by concussive wave propogating across the lung tissue interfaces.
b. Direct laceration of the lung by rib fracture.
c. Violent movement of chest wall leading to laceration of lung at sites of pleuroparenchymal adhesions.

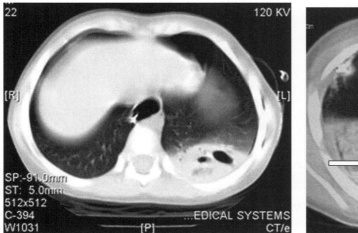 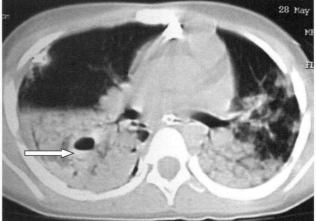

Figs 67A and B

CT FINDINGS

Seen as ovoid or elliptical lucencies with air-fluid levels often surrounded by contused lung parenchyma (arrow in Fig. 67B).

CASE 68

PULMONARY AV MALFORMATION

Abnormal vascular communication between a pulmonary artery and vein, or less commonly between systemic artery and pulmonary vein. May act as a low resistance right-left shunt. Isolated in 40%. Associated with Osler-Weber-Rendu diseases in upto 60%.

Three Types

- Single or few discrete AVF's
- Multiple discrete AVF's
- Multiple bilateral telangiectasias
  Single lesion found in 65% of cases.

Location—Anywhere, but usually lower lobes.

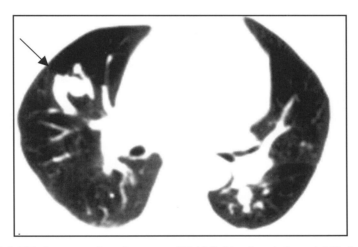

Fig. 68: Axial CT shows a simple type of PAVM in the right middle lobe (arrow)

CT demonstrates two types
1. Simple type—single feeding artery empties into a bulbous, segment with a single draining vein.
2. Complex type-more than one feeding artery and vein.

Seen as a Sharpley defined enhancing noncalcified nodule with an efferent vein. 70% in the lower lobes.

Complications—Stroke, brain abscess, hemoptysis, hemothorax.

VASCULAR CAUSES OF PULMONARY NODULES

1. **Atriovenous malformation**—Common from pulmonary artery to pulmonary vein
   Young female, lower lobe, most asymptomatic, 50% not associated with syndrome
   Shunt can allow systemic emboli, circle of Willis
   Angio—lolypop appearance dangling from artery, early drain vein

Usually well circumscribed, draining vein often visible, 60% solitary, multiple in case of hereditary telangiectasias.

CT—intense contrast enhancement unless thrombosed

Complications: Risk of systemic emboli, CVA, brain abscess and hemoptysis

2. **Pulmonary varix**—nonobstructive dilatation of pulm vein, dilation seen near L atrium, Assoc with Pulm venous HTN

3. Pulmonary artery aneurysm—congenital or aquired (Secondary to Swan-Ganz catheter injury, TB or mycotic aneurysms).

CASE 69

POLAND SYNDROME

Autosomal recessive disorder characterized by unilateral absence of sternocostal head of pectoralis major muscle. May be associated with ipsilateral syndactyly, brachydactyly or rib anomalies.

CT shows asymmetry of the chest wall with absence of pectoralis major muscle on the right side.

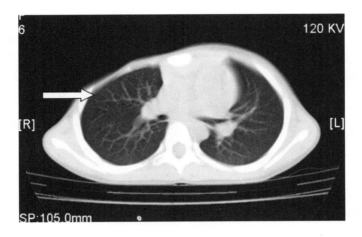

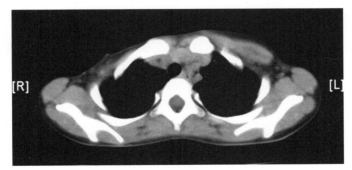

Figs 69A and B

CT FINDINGS

CT shows asymmetry of the chest wall with absence of pectoralis major muscle.

CASE 70

RASMUSSEN'S ANEURYSM

Pseudoaneurysm arising from the pulmonary artery resulting in inflammatory necrosis of the vessel. Most common cause is post primary tuberculosis. Typically the vessel injury occur in the upperlobes at sites of cavitary tuberculosis. Pathologically the terminal branches of PA are eroded within the walls.

Differential Diagnosis: Tuberculosis, aspergillosis, abscess, AVM, vasculitis, septic emboli.

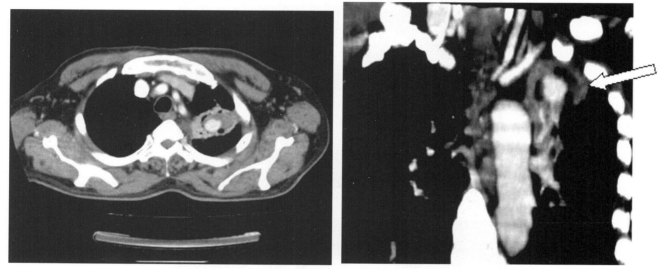

Figs 70A and B

CT FINDINGS

CT findings are an upper lobe parenchymal cavity with eccentric enhancing nodule and adjacent parenchymal fibrosis (arrow in Fig. 70B).

CASE 71

RETICULAR PATTERN

A reticular pattern consists of interlacing line shadows appearing as a mesh or net, and is associated with a heterogeneous group of interstitial lung diseases. These include idiopathic pneumonias (usual interstitial pneumonia [UIP], desquamative interstitial pneumonia [DIP], acute interstitial pneumonia [AIP], and nonspecific interstitial pneumonia [NSIP]); idiopathic pulmonary fibrosis (IPF); collagen vascular diseases; drug-induced lung disease; radiation pneumonitis and fibrosis; and asbestosis.

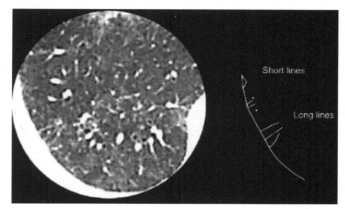

Fig. 71A

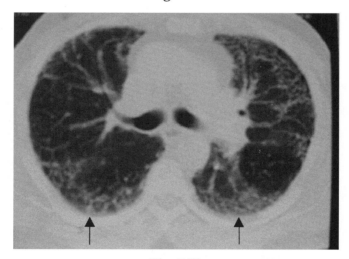

Fig. 71B

CT FINDINGS

CT lungs shows bilateral peripheral reticular opacities with areas of honeycombing (arrow).

CASE 72

ROUND ATELECTASIS

It is an unusual cause of pseudotumor known by many names characterized by the presence of a subpleural focus of airless lung.

- Atelectatic pseudotumor
- Pleuroma
- Folded lung syndrome
- Helical atelectasis
- Shrinking pleuritis with atelectasis
- Blesovsky syndrome

Pathogenesis

- Asbestos exposure causes pleural effusion with compressive atelectasis and parenchymal adherence to parietal pleura. With fluid resolution central lung re-expands and peripheral lung remains atelectatic
- Pleural fibrosis contracting with time with resultant compression of adjacent lung.

CT FINDINGS

- Rounded mass 3.5 to 7 cm.
- Subpleural location in a lower lobe
- Densest in periphery with air bronchogram in hilar aspect
- Contiguous pleural thickening
- Bronchovascular markings curve into the lesion
- Adjacent lung hyperinflated and oligemic.

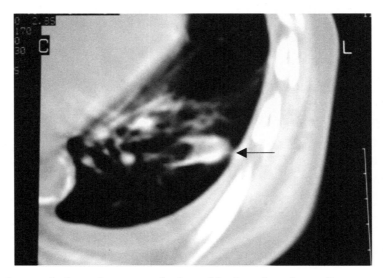

Fig. 72: Axial CT in lung window shows a subpleural lesion showing adjacent areas of hyperinflation and stretching of the bronchovascular markings (arrow)

CASE 73

RHEUMATOID LUNG

Rheumatoid arthritis is the most common of the connective tissue diseases, affecting about 1% of people worldwide. The disease can begin at any age, but the peak onset is in the fifth decade of life. The distribution of the arthritis usually is symmetric and diffuse. Women are affected two to three times more often than men. Although the most frequent clinical manifestation of RA is articular symptoms, extra-articular manifestations occur in more than three fourths of cases with severe involvement.

Although the ILD associated with RA is indistinguishable histologically from UIP, lung fibrosis usually is slowly progressive. Another form of interstitial pneumonia distinct from UIP, termed *nonspecific interstitial pneumonia*, may also occur in RA. This process is characterized by a diffuse lymphocyte and plasma cell infiltrate associated with relatively little fibrosis.

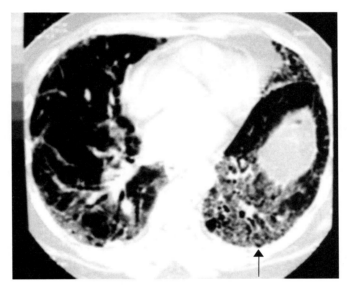

Fig. 73

High-resolution CT is much more sensitive than chest X-ray for the detection of early interstitial changes. **HRCT** depicts findings of fibrosis (i.e. interlobular septal thickening, traction bronchiectasis and bronchiolectasis, and honeycombing) and ground-glass opacity with a characteristic peripheral lower lobe predominance (Fig. 73). Other findings on CT include pleural thickening or effusion; small centrilobular nodules; and large nodular opacities (rheumatoid nodules).

RADIATION PNEUMONITIS

The prototype injury induced by radiation is called adhesive atelectasis due to absence of surfactant and may represent a form of resorptive atelectasis occurring without bronchial obstruction.

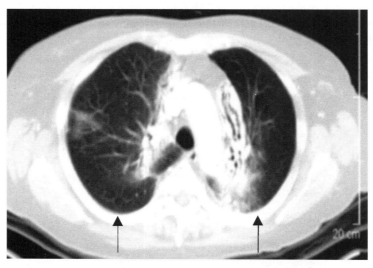

Fig. 74: Axial CT lungs shows bilateral paramediastinal ground glass attenuation with atelectasis in a patient who received radiation for lymphoma. Imaging changes are confined to the radiation field (arrows)

SILICOSIS

It is a fibrotic disease of the lung caused by inhalation of dust containing free crystalline silica. Three patterns of involvement is noted: 1) acute, 2) accelerated, and 3) chronic.

In patients with simple silicosis usually show well-defined nodules, 2-5 mm in diameter (range, 1-10 mm), that have an upper lobe and posterior lung zone predominance. Although silicosis and CWP are not easily distinguished by imaging methods, the nodules associated with silicosis tend to be more well-defined than those of CWP. In silicosis hilar lymphadenopathy may often be present, and may calcify in a peripheral pattern (so-called *"eggshell"* calcification) in 5% of cases.

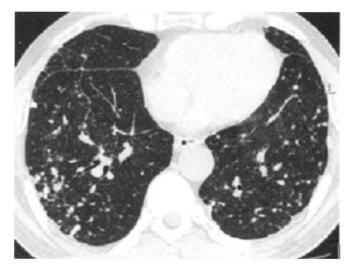

Fig. 75A: Axial HRCT reveals bilateral multiple centrilobular nodules in a Quarry worker

The development of opacities greater than 1 cm in diameter (usually in the upper lobes) on a background of small nodules indicates the presence of complicated silicosis. These opacities tend to migrate toward the hila, leaving irregular air space enlargement in their wake. Cavitation of these opacities suggests the diagnosis of tuberculosis.

HRCT findings of simple silicosis consists of small well-defined nodules in centrilobular distribution (sometimes in subpleural location). Nodules vary in size, usually ranging between 2-5 mm in diameter and may calcify.These nodules are predominantly seen in the posterior aspects of the upper lung zones and tend to be more widely and evenly distributed than nodules that are seen with sarcoidosis.

SILICO TUBERCULOSIS

Established silicosis is often associated with reactivation tuberculosis presenting as confluent consolidative opacities or cavitary changes. Other factors that may be predispose to reactivation TB include aging, malnutrition, uremia, diabetes, alcoholism.

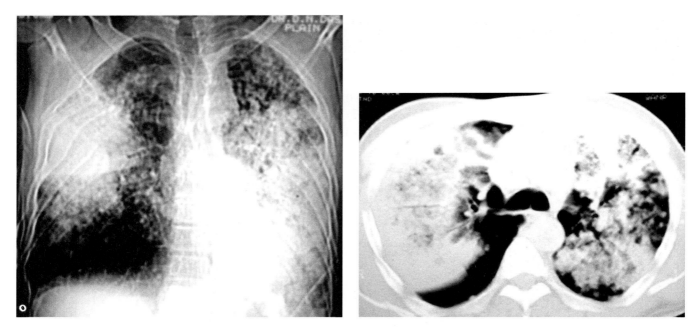

Figs 75B and C: (B) Digital scanogram shows bilateral upper and mid zone parenchymal infiltrates. (C) Axial CT shows bilateral parenchymal air space opacities with conglomeration seen in a 46-year-old male quarry worker who had previously documented subacute silicosis

SARCOIDOSIS

Sarcoidosis is a multisystem disorder of unknown etiology characterized by noncaseating granulomas. Affects patients between 20-40 years. Most of the morbidity and mortality is caused by pulmonary disease.

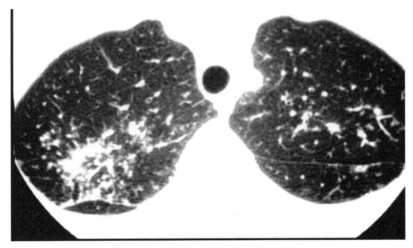

Fig. 76

Staging of sarcoid is done based on the pattern of involvement
Stage 0—clear chest X-ray.
Stage 1—node enlargement only.
Stage 2—nodes with parenchymal involvement.
Stage 3—parenchymal shadowing alone.

CT FINDINGS

- Characteristic findings consist of small nodules and nodular thickening along bronchovascular bundles, interlobular septa, interlobular fissures and subpleural lung regions (See Fig. 76).
- Thickening of bronchovascular interstitium is most marked in the perihilar regions of the upper and middle lung zones.
- Confluence of multiple small nodules may lead to large opacities ranging from 1-4 cm, some of which may have air bronchograms.
- Patchy areas of ground glass opacities can be seen.
- Late changes include fibrosis with irregular reticular opacities and altered lung architecture. Fibrosis leads to traction bronchiectasis and loss of lung volume.
- Honeycombing may also been seen in sarcoidosis. It is subpleural in location involving mainly middle and upper lung zones.
- Enlarged hilar and mediastinal nodes are present in 80-90% of patients,which may show calcification.

Differential Diagnosis

None of the radiographic or CT findings that can be produced by sarcoidosis are pathognomonic. The small nodules of sarcoidosis are characteristic, but small lung nodules similar to sarcoidosis are also common in lymphangitic lung metastases and silicosis. Lymphangitic metastases to the lung can closely resemble sarcoidosis. Small nodules distributed along lymphatics are common to both. Lymphangitic metastases, however, cause greater septal thickening and less distortion of the lobular anatomy than sarcoidosis. Silicosis is also characterized by small nodules and can look similar to sarcoidosis, but the history and clinical findings are distinctive.

SYSTEMIC SCLEROSIS (SCLERODERMA)

Progressive systemic sclerosis is an uncommon inflammatory-fibrotic disease of the skin (scleroderma) and some internal organs. Morbidity and mortality are related directly to the extent and severity of visceral involvement. The CREST syndrome is a limited form of scleroderma (subcutaneous calcinosis, Raynaud's phenomenon, esophageal dysmotility, sclerodactyly, and telangiectasia). Raynaud's phenomenon is the initial complaint in about 70% of patients. Similar changes occur in the vasculature of the heart, lung, kidneys, and gastrointestinal tract and contribute to the dysfunction of these organs.

The **HRCT** findings of interstitial fibrosis in PSS include ground-glass attenuation; subpleural reticular opacities; traction bronchiectasis and bronchiolectasis; architectural distortion; pleural thickening or effusion; and centrilobular micronodules (follicular bronchiolitis) in a predominantly peripheral and basilar distribution.

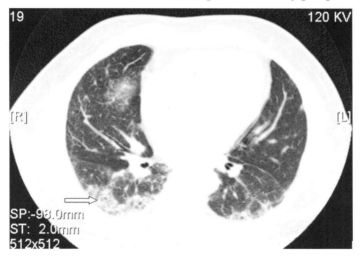

Fig. 77: Axial lung HRCT reveals bilateral basal subpleural ground glass attenuation (arrow) with reticular changes in a patient on treatment for scleroderma

CASE 78

SECONDARIES

Secondaries refer to the transport of viable tumour cells from one site of the body to another with respect to lungs metastasis can occur by four routes

1. Spread via pulmonary arteries.
2. Spread via pulmonary and pleural lymphatics.
3. Spread via airways.
4. Spread via pleural space

- Most common lung neoplasm
- In 15 to 25% of patients with lung metastases the lung is the only metastatic site
- Involve mainly the lower lung zones and frequently have peripheral distribution.

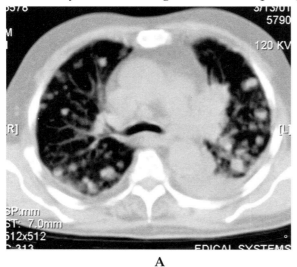
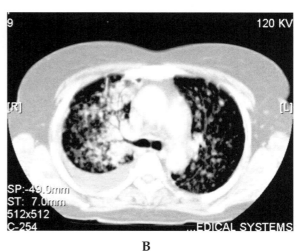

A   **B**

Figs 78A and B: (A) Axial CT lung shows bilateral multiple nodular opacities suggestive of secondaries in a patient with carcinoma stomach. (B) Axial CT lung shows bilateral nodular lesions along the bronchovascular and perilymphatic bundles in a patient with left lower lobe lung carcinoma

Common Primaries

- Breast
- Colon
- Pancreas
- Stomach
- Skin
- Head and neck
- Kidney

Pulmonary Metastases at Diagnosis of Primary Tumor

- Renal cell carcinoma
- Choriocarcinoma

- Wilms' tumor
- Ewing sarcoma
- Osteosarcoma

Mechanisms of Spread

- Hematogenous
- Lymphatic
- Direct extension
- Seeding of body cavities
- Transbronchial

CAVITATING METASTASES (4%) *(mnemonic Squamous Cell Metastases Tend to Cavitate)*

Squamous cell carcinoma, **S**arcoma
Colon
Melanoma
Transitional cell carcinoma
Cervix, under **C**hemotherapy

CALCIFYING METASTASES (<1%) *(mnemonic BOTTOM)*

Breast
Osteo-/chondrosarcoma
Thyroid (papillary)
Testicular
Ovarian
Mucinous adenocarcinoma

HEMORRHAGIC METASTASES

Choriocarcinoma
Renal cell carcinoma
Melanoma
Thyroid carcinoma

ENDOBRONCHIAL METASTASES

Bronchogenic carcinoma
Lymphoma
Renal cell carcinoma
Breast cancer
Colon carcinoma

CASE 79

SEPTAL THICKENING

An interlobular septum marginates part of a secondary pulmonary lobule and contains pulmonary veins and lymphatics. These septa measure approximately 0.1 mm in thickness and are occasionally seen on normal **HRCT** scans. Abnormal thickening of interlobular septa results from fibrosis, edema, or infiltration by cells or other material. Within the peripheral lung, thickened septa 1 to 2 cm in length may outline part or all of a secondary pulmonary lobule, perpendicular to the pleural surface. They represent the **HRCT** counterpart of Kerley's B lines seen on chest radiographs.

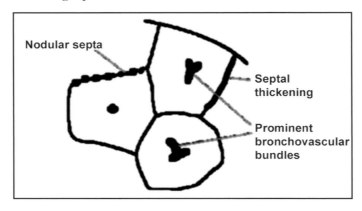

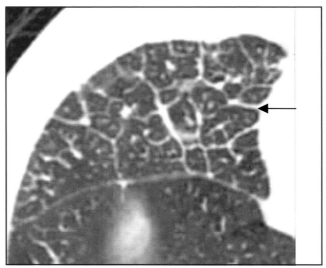

Fig. 79: Axial reconstructed lung section reveals septal thickening (arrow)

Interlobular septal thickening can be smooth, nodular, or irregular. Smooth thickening is seen in patients with pulmonary edema or hemorrhage, lymphangitic spread of carcinoma, lymphoma, leukemia, interstitial infiltration associated with amyloidosis, and some pneumonias. Nodular or beaded thickening occurs in lymphangitic spread of carcinoma or lymphoma, sarcoidosis, silicosis or coal workers' pneumoconiosis, lymphocytic interstitial pneumonia, and amyloidosis. Irregular thickening is seen in patients who have interstitial fibrosis.

CASE 80

SUBPLEURAL LINE

Thin curvilinear opacity parallel to and less than 1 cm from the pleura. May represent dependent opacity, but a subpleural line persisting in nondependent lung reflects fibrosis or honeycombing. These lines are thought to represent plate like atelectasis in the corticomedullary junction of the lung.

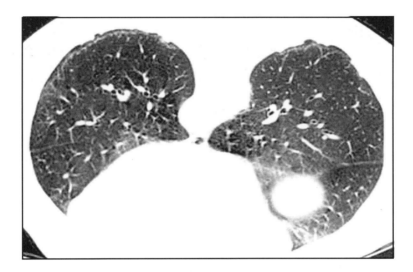

Fig. 80: Prone HRCT lung reveals bilateral subpleural persistant opacities suggestive of early fibrosis in a patient with restrictive lung disease

SOLITARY PULMONARY NODULE (SPN)

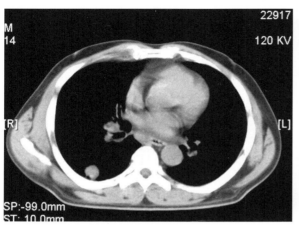 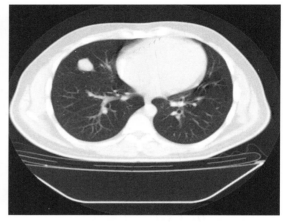

Figs 81A and B: (A) Shows a well marginated nodule in the right lowerlobe apical segment region peripherally. (B) Axial CT shows a nodule in the right middle lobe with lobulated margins–CT HU values and morphology is that of a indeterminate nodule

The Solitary Pulmonary Nodule: Approach, Differential Diagnosis, and Radiologic Evaluation

The solitary pulmonary nodule is a common radiologic abnormality that is often detected incidentally. Although most solitary pulmonary nodules have benign causes, many represent stage I lung cancers and must be distinguished from benign nodules in an expeditious and cost-effective manner.

Definitions

I. The following criteria must be met to classify a abnormality as a SPN:
   1. Round or oval lesion
   2. Circumscribed = surrounded by normal lung (although the borders may be sharp or ill-defined).
   3. Solitary
   4. No adenopathy or atelectasis
   5. Asymptomatic
   6. Size generally 1-6 cm (this is variable)
   7. No cavitation
   8. May or may not contain calcification.
II. Because the differential diagnosis of SPN is extensive, the major goal is to identify malignant nodules with as much certainty as possible and distinguish them from other causes of SPN that would not benefit from surgery. The differential diagnosis of the SPN is as follows:
   a. Malignancy:
      1. Primary pulmonary neoplasms:
         a. Bronchogenic carcinoma
         b. Lymphoma
         c. Carcinoid tumor
         d. Sarcoma, PNET, plasmacytoma

2. Secondary pulmonary neoplasms:
   a. Solitary metastasis: Renal, colon, breast, melanoma, testicular, sarcoma
3. Chest wall and pleural malignant neoplasms:
   a. Mesothelioma
   b. Pleural metastases
   c. Rib neoplasm: sarcoma, multiple myeloma, metastases

b. Benign pulmonary neoplasms and neoplastic-like conditions:
   1. Hamartoma
   2. Sclerosing hemangioma
   3. Intrapulmonary lymph node
   4. Mesenchymal neoplasms (**"oma's"**) (fibroma, chondroma, granular cell myoblastoma, hemangiopericytoma, neurofibroma, leiomyoma, lipoma, chemodectoma)
   5. Clear cell ("sugar") tumor
   6. Pulmonary hyalinizing granuloma
   7. Plasma cell granuloma
   8. Amyloid
   9. Paraffinoma (lipoid pneumonia)

c. Infections:
   1. Mycobacteria (particularly MTB)
   2. Fungi: coccidiomycosis, histoplasmosis, aspergillus, cryptococcus
   3. Nocardia
   4. Pyogenic pneumonia ("round" pneumonias), abscess
   5. Parasites (esp. *Echinococcus*, dog heartworm, hookworm, *Ascaris*)
   6. Virus: measles

d. Non-parenchymal causes:
   1. Chest wall lesions:
      a. Artifacts: nipple, mole, ECG leads
      b. Skin/breast tumor (including neurofibromas in NF)
      c. Rib lesions: fracture, osteochondroma
      d. Pleural lesions: loculated fluid, focal fibrous tumor of the pleura, fibrin ball

e. Vascular causes:
   1. AVM
   2. Aneurysm of pulmonary artery
   3. Varix
   4. Anomalous pulmonary vein
   5. Infarct.

f. Trauma: hematoma

g. Non-infectious inflammatory:
   1. Wegener's granulomatosis
   2. Rheumatoid
   3. Sarcoid
   4. Organizing pneumonia
   5. Pneumoconiosis

h. Airway causes:
   1. Bronchial atresia

    2. Bronchocele
    3. Infected/fluid filled bulla
  i. Congenital:
    1. Bronchogenic cyst
    2. Sequestration
  j. Other:
    1. Endometriosis
    2. Extramedullary hematopoiesis
    3. Talc granuloma.

Appearance of SPN on CT Scanning

1. CT scanning provides better assessment of the borders of a lesion. Air bronchograms may be more easily seen within a lesion on CT scanning, and are more likely seen in malignancy than benign etiologies of SPNs.
2. CT scanning more effectively demonstrates the presence of additional nodules.
3. CT is the only way to preoperatively reveal fat in hamartomas.
4. CT scanning may demonstrate other scan findings of relevance (e.g. adenopathy)
5. CT may reveal satellite lesions, which tend to favor a benign diagnosis
a. *Presence and pattern of calcification:* CT is more sensitive for the demonstration of calcification within SPNS; it may reveal calcification in about 25% of nodules that were not definitely calcified on plain films or tomograms.
b. *Benign patterns of calcification include:*
    1. Diffuse calcification
    2. Laminar calcification
    3. Central/target calcification
    4. "Popcorn/chondroid" calcification
c. *Patterns of calcification, which are not definitely benign, are:*
    1. Speckled calcification
    2. Eccentric calcification- this situation may occur when a granuloma is engulfed by an adjacent carcinoma.
d. *Two circumstances must be remembered:*
    1. Carcinoid tumors may calcify densely
    2. Osteogenic sarcoma metastases may calcify densely.

CT is helpful in detecting other nodules not apparent on chest X-ray and in biopsy planning.

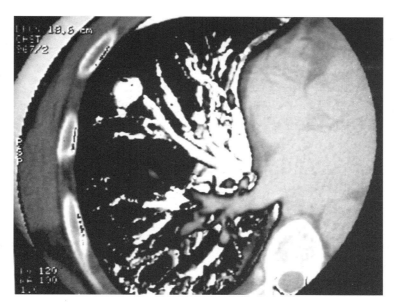

Fig. 81C: 3D surface shaded display of peripheral nodule for volume estimation (same case as in Fig. 81B)

Factors of Malignant vs Benign SPN		
	Malignant	*Benign*
Size	Large	Small
Calcium	Eccentric or stippled	Diffuse, central, laminated, or popcorn
Smoking Hx	Present	Absent
Age	Elderly	<35 years
2 × time	20-400 days	> 450 or < 20 days

CASE 82

SEQUESTRATION

- No normal communication to the tracheobronchial tree
  - Systemic blood supply
- Extralobar sequestration
  - Invested in its own pleura
- Intralobar sequestration
  - Shares the pleura of the parent lung
- ILS: ELS 4:1

Extralobar Sequestration (ELS)

Pathogenesis

- Abnormal budding from foregut or tracheobronchial tree
- Induction of pulmonary mesenchyma into formation of lung parenchyma
- Sequestered in its own pleural investment and without normal communication to the tracheobronchial tree
- Persistence of systemic blood supply
- Left sided - 65-90%
- Location:
  - Between lower lobe and diaphragm - 63%
  - Intradiaphragmatic
  - Mediastinal
  - Abdominal
- Arterial supply—Systemic
  - Aorta (80%), other arteries
  - Rarely pulmonary
- Venous drainage—Systemic (80%)
  - Occasionally to pulmonary veins

CT FINDINGS (Fig. 82A)

- Triangular/rounded soft tissue mass or consolidation
- Systemic vascular supply
  - Systemic venous drainage

Intralobar Sequestration (ILS)

Clinical

- Males = Females
- Symptomatic in >50% of patients by age 20
- Cough, sputum production, and recurrent pneumonia
- First complaints rarely seen after age 50

Intralobar Sequestration

- - 5%

CT FINDINGS (Fig. 82B)

- Infiltrate, mass, ill-defined density
  - Recurrent pneumonia
  - Posterior basal segment lower lobe
- Solid, cystic, air-fluid levels
- Systemic arterial supply

Pulmonary venous drainage	
ELS	*ILS*
Own pleura	Shared pleura
60% under 1 year	50% after 20 years
90% left	60% left
M:F 4:1	M:F 1:1
Solid	Cystic or Solid
Systemic arterial supply	Systemic arterial supply
Systemic venous drainage	Pulmonary venous drainage

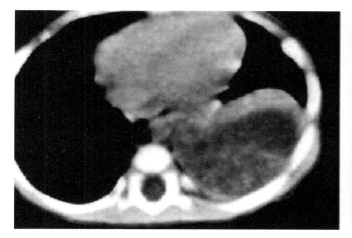 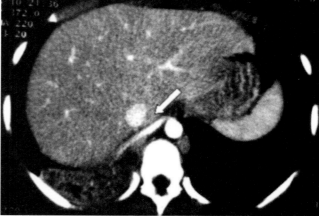

Figs 82A and B: (A) Axial CT in mediastinal window shows a lower lobe heterogenous opacity causing compressive atelectasis of underlying lung. (B) Axial CT with contrast reveals right lower zone heterogenous opacity showing an aberrant blood supply from the aorta (arrow)

TRACHEOMEGALY

May be primary –Mounier-Kuhn syndrome characterized by dysplasia of cartilage of trachea and major bronchi with abrupt transition to normal dimension at 5th order bronchi.

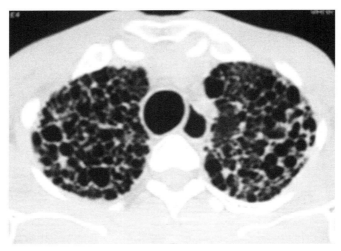

Fig. 83: Axial CT lungs shows tracheomegaly with conglomerate cystic changes involving both the lung fields

Secondary tracheobronchomegaly may result as a sequlae to fibrosis, or end stage lung disease. Usual age of presentation is 3-5th decade, present with recurrent lower respiratory infection and shortness of breathe.
CT shows enlarged trachea > 29 mm, enlarged right main bronchus >20 mm, left main bronchus >15 mm.

CASE 84

TRACTION BRONCHIECTASIS

Irregular bronchiectasis occurring due to traction of fibrous tissue on the bronchial walls. Seen in pulmonary fibrosis of varied etiology.

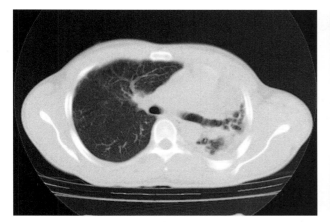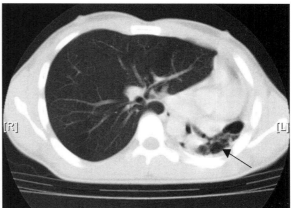

Figs 84A and B: Axial CT lungs show left lung volume loss with traction ectasia of segmental and lobar bronchi (arrow)

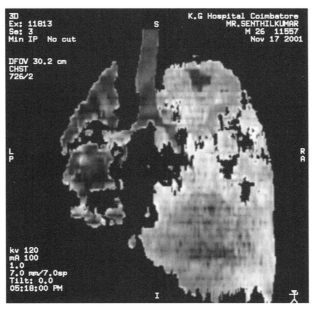

Fig. 84C: Minimum intensity projection shows the traction ectactic changes as black areas in both lungs, more on the right side

CASE 85

TRANSBRONCHIAL SPREAD

Seen usually in infectious diseases as multiple nodular opacities suggestive of impacted bronchioles. Commonly seen in cavitary Kochs diseases due to spread to adjacent segment due to repeated aspirations.

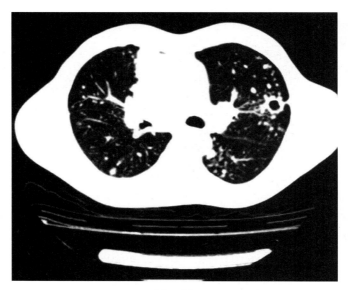

Fig. 85

CT FINDINGS

CT shows left upper lobe cavitary lesion with multiple bilateral nodular opacities due to bronchiolar impaction. In a case of primary Koch's disease.

CASE 86

TUBERCULOSIS

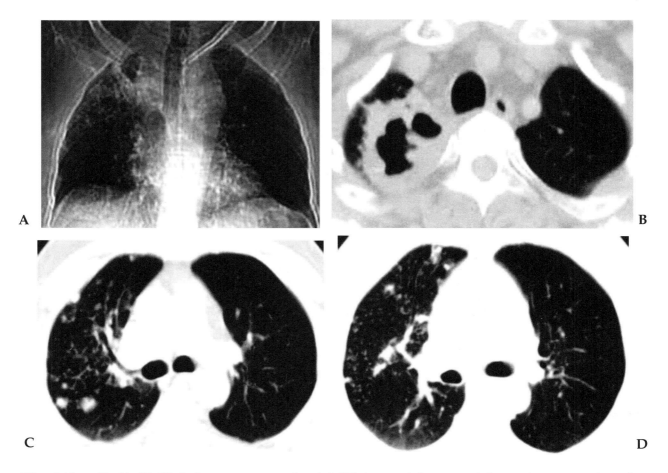

Figs 86A to D: (A, B) Digital scanogram and axial CT shows right upper lobe cavity suggestive of active post-primary Koch's lesion in 36 year old male alcoholic patient. (C, D) Axial CT in a 23 year old female shows multiple nodules suggestive of transbronchial spread

Pathogenesis

- Droplet inhalation (2 to 10 um/1 to 3 bacilli)
  - Bacilli deposited in mid/lower lung
  - Ghon focus 1 - 2 cm
- Interaction with lymphocytes/macrophages
  - Regional nodal spread - Ghon complex
  - Lymphatic and hematogenous spread
- Immunity - 6 to 10 weeks
  - Intracellular killing of bacilli and healing
- Release of hydrolytic enzymes
  - Caseation, fibrosis, calcification

-157-

Hematogenous Dissemination

- Areas of high oxygen tension
  - Subapical upper lobe
  - Epiphysis of long bones
  - Brain
  - Renal cortex
- Apical and posterior segments
  - Decreased perfusion in upright position
  - Decreased lymphatic flow and clearance
- Subapical nodules
  - Healing with scar formation
  - Surrounding overexpanded air spaces
- Little or no host response - Miliary TB

Tuberculosis

Clinical
- Primary
  - Asymptomatic - 90%
  - Symptomatic pneumonia
  - Progressive primary tuberculosis
  - Cough, hemoptysis, weight loss
- Postprimary
  - Chronic cough
  - Weight loss
  - Occasional hemoptysis, dyspnea
  - May be asymptomatic

Primary Tuberculosis

Children
- Most common form of disease
- Asymptomatic
- Non-specific signs and symptoms
- Occasionally acute illness with fever, chest pain, and consolidation

Primary Childhood TB

Radiologic Findings
- Hilar lymphadenopathy, usually unilateral
- Consolidation
- Right side more commonly involved
  - Atelectasis - middle lobe
  - Cavitation of parenchymal component
- Pleural effusion
- Miliary tuberculosis
  - Within 6 months of primary infection

Primary Tuberculosis

Radiologic Findings

- Consolidation
  - Mid/lower lung, anterior segment, upper lobe
  - Failure to clear with antibiotics
  - Cavitation
- Lymphadenopathy (10 - 40%)
  - Hilar and/or mediastinal
- Pleural effusion (10%)
  - Unilateral, large, exudate
- Lobar atelectasis
- Miliary disease (2 to 6%), 2 mm nodules throughout lung
  - CT—Sharply or poorly defined, Intra or interlobular

Postprimary Tuberculosis

- Long after initial exposure
- Reactivation of dormant foci of infection
- Chronic, slowly progressive
- Acute necrotizing pneumonia in upper lung with cavitation (3 - 10 cm)
  - Early cavities—thin walls
  - Chronic cavities—thick fibrous walls

Radiologic Findings

- Upper lobe—apical/posterior
- Chronic consolidation
- Cavitation common (45%)
  - Air fluid levels
  - Solitary/Multiple
  - Thick or thin walls
- Volume loss, bronchiectasis, bronchostenosis
- Endobronchial spread (20%)
  - Multiple small acinar shadows
  - Dependent portions of lung
  - Progression to confluent disease
- Pleural disease
  - Effusion, Tuberculous empyema
  - Spontaneous pneumothorax (5%)
- Nodule or mass (tuberculoma)
  - Solitary or multiple - 0.5 - 4.0 cm
  - Round or oval, well marginated
  - Satellite lesions (80%)

Tuberculosis

Complications
- End stage lung disease
- Fatal hemoptysis 1-5%
- Rasmussen aneurysm
  - Weakening of arterial wall from cavitary TB (see Case 70)
- Aspergilloma
- Chest wall involvement - Osseous destruction.

TREE-IN-BUD

The CT pattern of centrilobular nodular and branching linear opacities has been likened to the appearance of a tree-in-bud. Many disorders can result in this pattern, the most common being infectious processes with endobronchial spread of disease. The common CT features of all processes producing the tree-in-bud pattern are bronchiolar dilatation, and impaction of bronchioles with mucus, pus, or other material. The CT findings are nonspecific, but a specific diagnosis can occasionally be suggested when the findings are correlated with patient history, clinical information, associated CT scan findings, and chronicity of disease.

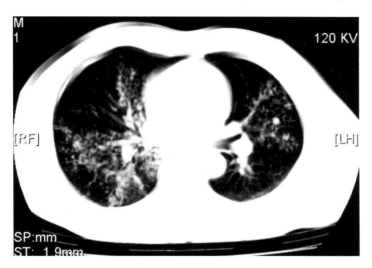

Fig. 87

The term *tree-in-bud* dates back to the bronchogram descriptions of normal respiratory bronchioles by Twining and Kerley to describe the CT appearance of the endobronchial spread of *Mycobacterium tuberculosis*.

Tree-in-bud: Differential Diagnosis

Infection

Allergic bronchopulmonary aspergillosis

Cystic fibrosis

Aspiration

Diffuse panbronchiolitis

Obliterative bronchiolitis

Asthma

THREE DIMENSIONAL RENDERING TECHNIQUES

Progressive improvements in helical CT scanners over the past few years have greatly revolutionized the performance of thoracic CT studies. Multidimensional imaging with near isotropic voxels and fewer artifacts is possible with these new scanners. Computer hardware has similarly improved such that a three-dimensional image. This allows for more precise vascular imaging and can provide surgeons exquisite anatomic data for surgical planning. Within the lung, the tracheobronchial tree can be mapped, pulmonary nodules can be detected and categorized more readily, and lung volumes can be measured precisely.

IMAGING TECHNIQUES

Two-dimensional Multiplanar Reconstruction

Two-dimensional multiplanar and curved reformations (MPR) help solve the inherent difficulties of assessing the craniocaudal extent of disease on axial images. By changing the plane in which this volumetric data is displayed, two-dimensional reformatted images can be produced in the coronal and sagittal planes, any obliquity can be obtained to display best the long axis of the region in question. However, it is important to review the source axial images because artifact along the Z axis can occur and result in misdiagnosis.

Three-dimensional Maximum and Minimum Intensity Projection

Maximum (MIP) and minimum intensity projection (minIP) images are created in a similar fashion. Three-dimensional images are obtained by passing parallel rays through the volume data and displaying only the highest (or lowest) attenuation voxels. Because only select voxels are used, over 95% of the original data are lost. MIP and minIP images have a tendency to misrepresent spatial relationships and are of limited use in areas of complex vascular anatomy and overlapping structures.

Three-dimensional Shaded Surface Display and Volume Rendering

Three-dimensional shaded surface display (SSD) rendering techniques have been largely replaced by volume rendering. Three-dimensional SSD uses a range of attenuation values to define surfaces and create an image. Anatomic accuracy is dependent on the imaging parameters chosen.

Three-dimensional volume rendering has the advantage of using all of the data in creating the final image. Each voxel is summed and displayed as a composite image on the monitor. By choosing different parameters the data can be segmented by attenuation values to display the desired structure, such as the airway, blood vessels, or chest wall. Because volume rendering is less user-dependent, measurement of vascular or airway stenoses, particularly in those structures perpendicular to the axial plane, is more accurately obtained. By changing the opacity and shading characteristics, one can "see through" closer structures to those further away. Volume rendering can be performed from an internal perspective allowing the user to "fly through" hollow structures.

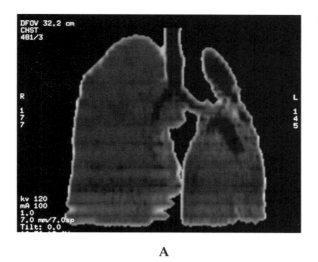

A

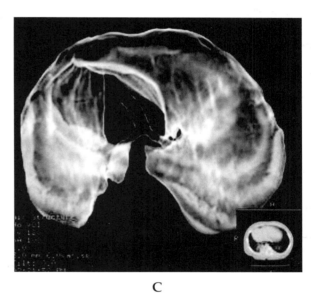

B   C

Figs 88A to C: (A) Minimum intensity projection highlights air useful for imaging of trachea. (B) Surface rendering (SSD) is useful for studying the external morphological alteration of lung diseases. (C) Most useful rendering technique to visualize all structures in the region of interest

CASE 89

WEGENER'S GRANULOMA

Wegener's Granulomatosis

Necrotizing granuloma of upper and lower airways caused by vasculitis of arteries and veins first described by Wegener in 1936.

Clinical Presentation

- Classic triad: sinusitis, pulmonary symptoms and renal insufficiency
- Onset and course extremely variable
- Chronic upper respiratory tract symptoms may persist for years before pulmonary disease
- May present as overwhelming diffuse vasculitis

Earliest Lesions: Bilateral Reticulo-nodular Opacities

- Bilateral multifocal nodules: 5 mm-10 cm
- Sharply marginated
- Cavitation 20-50%
- Evolve from thick walls to thin walled cysts with treatment
- Airspace consolidation.
- Predominant subpleural location
- Cavitation in nodules greater than 2cm
- Feeding vessels enter nodules (88%)
- Pleural based lesions mimic infarcts
- CT "halo sign"

Airway Involvement

- Endobronchial abnormalities (59% bronchoscopy)
- Subglottic stenosis
- Ulcerating tracheobronchitis
- Tracheal or bronchial stenosis
- Often multifocal with variable length of involvement
- CT key for evaluation, chest X-ray often normal

Lab Parameters to be evaluated:

- Serum Antineutrophil Cytoplasmic Autoantibody (ANCA)
- c-ANCA cytoplasmic pattern, reacts with proteinase 3
- 99% specificity and 96% sensitivity in generalized active disease
- c-ANCA positivity drops to 30% in remission
- p-ANCA perinuclear pattern, reacts with myeloperoxidase
- p-ANCA positive in collagen vascular diseases

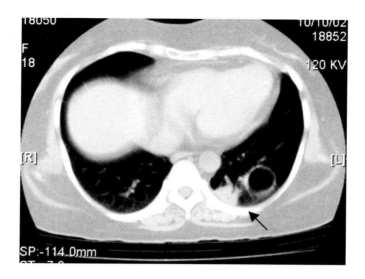

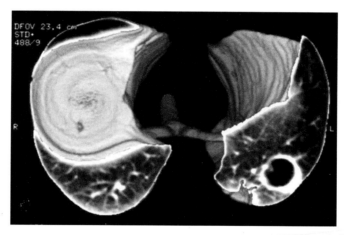

Figs 89A and B: Axial CT with surface shaded 3D lung rendering (89B) reveals a left lower lobe cavitary lesion with adjacent patchy consolidation (arrow). Patient is a known case of Wegener's on follow up. Previous CT scan showed a homogenous opacity at the site of the cavity

CASE 90

SIGNS IN THORACIC CT

AIR BRONCHOGRAM SIGN

This sign refers to one or more linear or branching tubular but tapering lucencies representing bronchi or bronchioles passing through densely opacified lung parenchyma. An air bronchogram within an opacity confirms that the opacity is intrapulmonary, not pleural or mediastinal, in location.

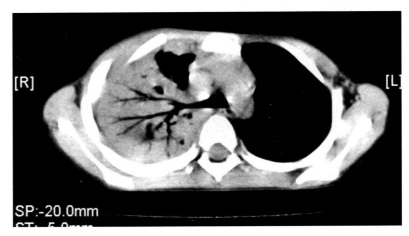

Fig. 90

The most common causes of an air bronchogram are pneumonia and certain neoplasms. Although cancers tend to be solid masses, lymphoma and bronchoalveolar cell carcinoma are characteristically associated with the air bronchogram sign.

AIR CRESCENT SIGN

A tumor or fungal mass growing within a pre-existing cavity, or an area of pneumonia that undergoes necrosis and cavitates, can form a peripheral crescent of air between the intracavitary mass and the cavity wall, resulting in the air crescent sign.

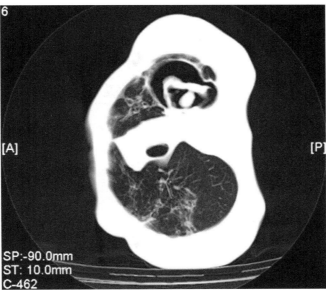

Fig. 91

A tumor or fungal mass growing within a pre-existing cavity, or an area of pneumonia that undergoes necrosis and cavitates, can form a peripheral crescent of air between the intracavitary mass and the cavity wall, resulting in the air crescent.

DROWNED LUNG SIGN

This sign refers to gas absorption and replacement of air by edema fluid distal to an acute bronchial obstruction. On CT, the bronchi within the lobe are prominently visualized because they are filled with low-attenuation material, yielding a mucus bronchogram.

This sign is similar to, and may be seen with, the CT angiogram and air bronchogram signs. If the obstruction persists and the obstructed lobe remains sterile, excess edema fluid and blood within the drowned lobe are gradually reabsorbed. The affected lobe enlarges when there is a buildup of secretions and infection behind the obstructing lesion, often seen in postobstructive pneumonia related to endobronchial carcinoma.

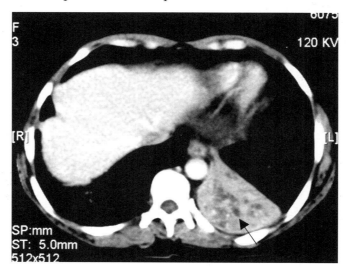

Fig. 92

FALLEN LUNG SIGN

The fallen lung refers to a diagnostic but uncommon CT sign of complete or near complete bronchial transection, in which the collapsed lung falls away from the hilum toward the lateral and posterior chest wall or diaphragm with supine positioning. Normally, the lung collapses inward toward the hilum. The finding is usually associated with a large pneumothorax, which because of the free communication between the fractured airway and the pleural space, is persistent despite thoracostomy tube drainage. Pneumomediastinum is also commonly seen. CT may directly show the bronchial tear as discontinuity or focal narrowing of the affected bronchus.

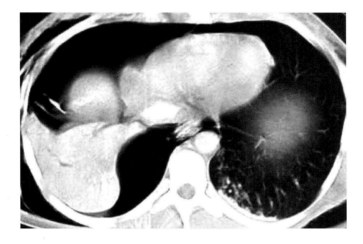

Fig. 93

GLOVED FINGER SIGN

This sign is characteristically seen when central bronchi are involved with allergic bronchopulmonary aspergillosis, a clinical disorder secondary to aspergillus hypersensitivity. In this case, the bronchi become impacted with mucus, cellular debris, eosinophils, and fungal hyphae. This sign can also be seen in cystic fibrosis, another disease in which central bronchiectasis predominates

When bronchiectatic segments become filled with mucus or pus, they appear on CT as opacities with distinctive shapes, variously described as gloved finger, finger-in-glove, Y, V, inverted V, toothpaste.

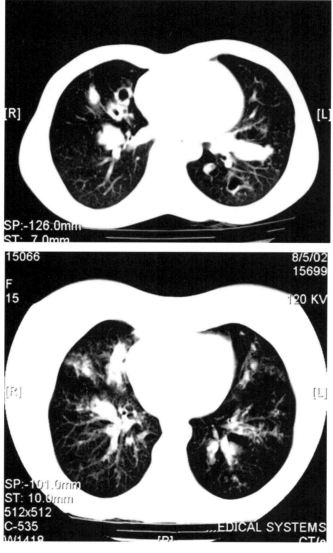

Figs 94A and B

CASE 95

GOLDEN 'S' SIGN

When a lobe collapses around a large central mass, the peripheral lung collapses and the central portion of lung is prevented from collapsing by the presence of the mass. The affected fissure has a central convexity because of the mass itself and distal concavity as a result of atelectasis, resembling an S or a reverse S shape.

Initially described for right upper lobe atelectasis, the sign is applicable to atelectasis of any lobe. The importance of this sign is to realize the presence of central obstruction. In an adult, an underlying bronchogenic carcinoma is usually the cause of obstruction.

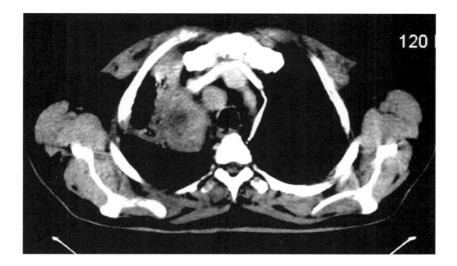

Fig. 95

CASE 96

HALO SIGN

This CT scan sign refers to GGO surrounding or forming a halo around a denser nodule or focal area of consolidation.

Hemorrhagic pulmonary nodules, such as those seen with Kaposi's sarcoma metastases, metastatic angiosarcoma, Wegener's granulomatosis, and infection from Candida species, Mucorales species, cytomegalovirus, and herpes simplex can produce this sign. When seen in patients with acute leukemia, the halo sign is highly suggestive of early angioinvasive pulmonary aspergillosis. In this case, the halo is related to the presence of hemorrhage surrounding the central necrotic nodule. With time, these lesions may develop air crescents and progress to frank cavitation.

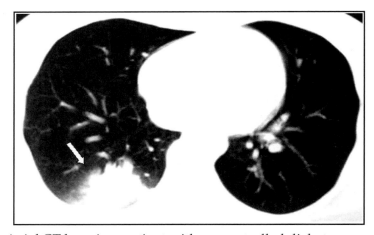

Fig. 96: Axial CT lung in a patient with uncontrolled diabetes reveals a right lower lobe parenchymal opacity with a peripheral marginal halo (arrow)

CASE 97

HAMPTON'S HUMP SIGN

Pulmonary infarction secondary to pulmonary embolism produces an abnormal area of opacification on the chest radiograph or CT scan, which is always in contact with the pleural surface. The opacification usually resembles a truncated cone, so-called *Hampton's hump.*

The configuration of the opacity is that of homogeneous wedge-shaped consolidation in the lung periphery, with the base contiguous to a visceral pleural surface and the rounded, convex apex directed toward the hilum. The size of the consolidated area varies, usually 3 to 5 cm in diameter but reaching 10 cm. Air bronchograms are rarely seen. When necrosis occurs, radiologic clearing may take weeks. The pattern of resolution is a helpful indicator of pulmonary infarction, which gradually diminishes while maintaining its homogenity and original shape the so-called *melting ice cube sign.*

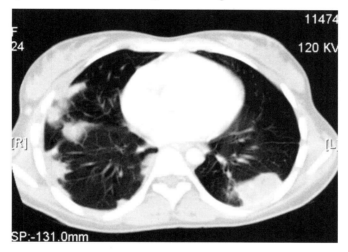

Fig. 97

CASE 98

CT ANGIOGRAM SIGN

The CT angiogram sign is caused by the homogeneous low attenuation of consolidation, which allows vessels to be seen clearly particularly after intravenous administration of contrast material. The CT angiogram sign is nonspecific and also may be seen in lobar pneumonia, pulmonary lymphoma lipid pneumonia, pulmonary infarction, and pulmonary edema.

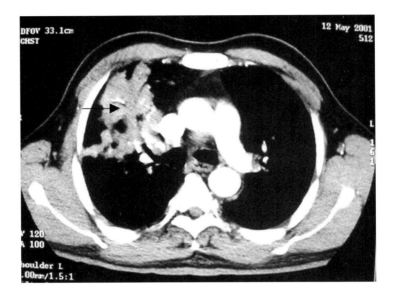

Fig. 98

SIGNET-RING SIGN

Ring shadow (representing dilated thick-walled bronchus) with small soft tissue opacity (representing adjacent pulmonary artery) in its periphery diagnostic of bronchiectasis.

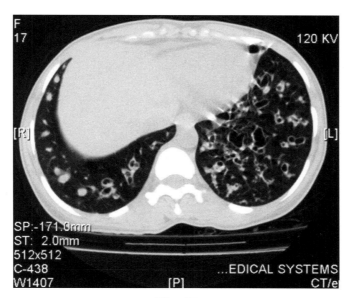

Fig. 99

SPLIT PLEURA SIGN

Normally, the thin visceral and parietal pleura cannot be distinguished as two separate structures on CT scanning. With empyema, the fluid separates or splits the thickened and contrast-enhancing pleural.

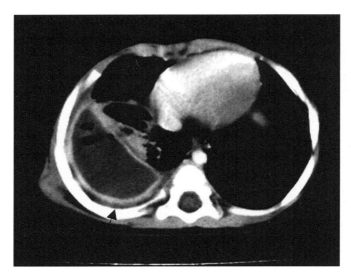

Fig. 100

The split pleura sign allows confident distinction of loculated empyema from a peripheral lung abscess. Other processes that lead to pleuritis, such as hemothorax and treatment of malignant pleural effusion with talc pleurodesis, can also result in this appearance on CT.

CT FINDINGS

- Lenticular shape
- Obtuse angle with chest wall
- Walls of uniform thickness
- Smooth inner and outer margins
- Split pleura sign/Separation of the pleural layers (see Fig.)
- Compression of adjacent lung

CASE 101

WESTERMARK SIGN

This sign refers to focal oligemia of the lung distal to an occluded pulmonary artery. Oligemia distal to an obstructing embolus, so-called *Westermark sign*, is a relatively uncommon finding.

Bronchial obstruction is not a feature, there is no overinflation and lung volume may be reduced. A similar CT appearance of lung oligemia may be produced by neoplastic obstruction of a pulmonary artery secondary to either invasion by a contiguous carcinoma or intravascular growth of a primary sarcoma.

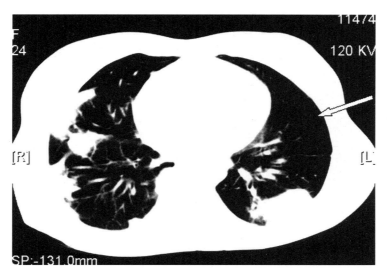

Fig. 101. Axial CT shows multiple peripheral parenchymal infarcts, left lingula shows paucity of vascular markings (arrow)

CASE 102

LUFTSICHEL SIGN

In upper lobe collapse, there is hyperinflation of the superior segment of the lower lobe. This hyperinflated lung is seen as a crescent-shaped lucency called a *luftsichel*, derived from the German words "luft" (air) and "sichel" (sickle). This sign is more often seen on the left side, in which the hyperinflated superior segment of the left lower lobe is positioned between the aortic arch and the collapsed left upper lobe. CT shows a V-shaped or peaked appearance of the posteromedial fissural surface between the atelectatic upper lobe and the overinflated lower lobe segment. This sign, and associated findings of upper lobe collapse, signify the diagnosis of an endobronchial mass, such as endobronchial carcinoma.

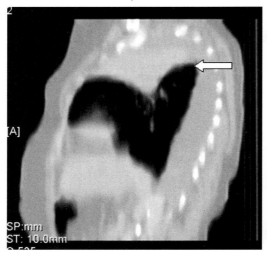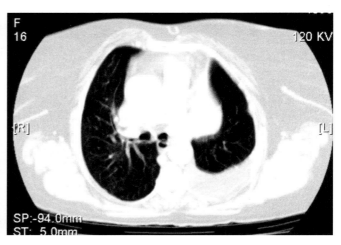

Fig. 102

Appendix
Compilation of Useful Hints
for Chest Imaging

Predilection of Diseases

Upper Lobe

1. S—Silicosis (progressive massive fibrosis)
   Sarcoidosis
2. C—Coal workers pneumoconiosis
3. H—Histiocytosis X
4. A—Ankylosing spondylitis, aspergillosis
5. R—Radiation
6. T—TB

Lower Lobe

1. R—Rheumatoid arthritis
2. A—Asbestosis
3. S—Scleroderma
4. I—Idiopathic
5. O—Other
   —Busulphan, bleomycin, amiodarone, methotrexate

Diffuse Interstitial Disease + Mediastinal Lymphadenopathy

1. Carcinoma
2. Lymphoma
3. Sarcoidosis
4. Silicosis
5. Viral infection

Diffuse Interstitial Disease + Skeletal Abnormality

1. Ribs—Scleroderma
2. Spine—Ankylosing spondylitys
3. Shoulder joints—RA, scleroderma, sarcoidosis
   —hypertrophic pulmonary osteoarthropathy
4. Skull—Tuberous sclerosis, histiocytosis X

Diagnostic Thinking—Deriving the Differential Diagnosis

A. System/Structure-Related
   1. Cardiovascular
   2. Pulmonary
   3. Neurologic
   4. Etc.
B. Process-Related
   1. Vascular and cardiac
   2. Infectious/Inflammatory
   3. Neoplastic
   4. Degenerative
   5. Intoxication/Iatrogenic/Idiopathic

6. **Congenital**
7. **Autoimmune/Allergic**
8. **Trauma**
9. **Endocrine**

EXTRAPULMONARY PHYSICAL FINDINGS IN INTERSTITIAL LUNG DISEASE	
Systemic hypertension	Connective tissue disease, neurofibromatosis, diffuse alveolar hemorrhage syndromes
Erythema nodosum	Sarcoidosis, connective tissue disease, Behcet's syndrome
Maculopapular rash	Drug induced, amyloidosis, lipoidosis, connective tissue disease, Gauchers disease
Heliotrope rash	Dermatomyositis
Albinism	Hermansky-Pudlak syndrome
Discoid lupus	Idiopathic pulmonary fibrosis, systemic lupus erythematosus
Neurofibroma	von Recklinghausen's disease
Telangiectasia	Scleroderma
Raynaud's phenomena	Idiopathic pulmonary fibrosis, connective tissue disease
Cutaneous vasculitis	Systemic vasculitides, connective tissue disorders
Subcutaneous nodules	von Recklinghausen's disease, rheumatoid arthritis
Calcinosis	Dermatomyositis, scleroderma
Uveitis	Sarcoidosis, Behcet's syndrome, ankylosing spondylitis
Scleritis	Systemic vasculitis, systemic lupus erythematosus, scleroderma, sarcoidosis
Keratoconjunctivitis sicca	Lymphocytic interstitial pneumonia
Salivary gland enlargement	Sarcoidosis, lymphocytic interstitial pneumonia
Peripheral lympadenopathy	Sarcoidosis, lymphangitic carcinomatosis, lymphocytic interstitial pneumonia, lymphoma
Hepatosplenomegaly	Sarcoidosis, eosinophilic granuloma, connective tissue disease, amyloidosis, lymphocytic interstitial pneumonia
Pericarditis	Radiation pneumonitis, connective tissue disease
Myositis	Connective tissue disease, drugs (L-tryptophan)
Bone involvement	Sarcoidosis, eosinophilic granuloma, Gaucher's disease, lymphangitic carcinomatosis
Arthritis	Connective tissue disease, systemic vasculitis, sarcoidosis
Diabetes insipidus	Eosinophilic granuloma, sarcoidosis
Glomerulonephritis	Systemic vasculitis, connective tissue disease, Goodpasture's syndrome, sarcoidosis
Nephrotic syndrome	Amyloidosis, drug induced (gold, pencillamine), systemic lupus erythematosus

Features	AIP	UIP	NSIP	BOOP
Contrasting Clinical, Radiologic, and Histologic Features of AIP, UIP, NSIP, and BOOP*				
	Clinical			
Mean age, yr	49	57	49	56
Sex, M/F†	No predilection	1.8:1	1:1.4	No predilection
Onset	Acute	Insidious	Subacute, insidious	Subacute
Symptoms	Dyspnea, respiratory failure	Dyspnea, cough	Dyspnea, cough	Dyspnea, cough
Mortality rate (mean survival)	62% (1-2 mo)	68% (5-6 yr)	11% (17 mo)	6% (< 4 mo)
Response to steroids	Poor	Poor	Good	Good
Complete recovery possible	Yes	No	Yes	Yes
	Radiologic			
Chest radiograph	Bilateral diffuse airspace opacities	Bilateral interstitial reticulonodular infiltrates, honeycomb changes, accentuation in lung bases	Bilateral interstitial infiltrates	Bilateral patchy opacities
HRCT scans	Bilateral diffuse ground-glass attenuation	Same as above	Bilateral patchy ground-glass attenuation	Same as above
	Pathologic			
Temporal appearance	Uniform	Heterogeneous	Uniform	Uniform
Interstitial inflammation	Scant	Scant	Usually prominent	Variable
Collagen fibrosis	No	Patchy	Variable, diffuse	No
Fibroblast proliferation	Diffuse, interstitial	Patchy (fibroblast foci)	Occasional	Patchy, air space
BOOP areas	Rare	No	Rare	—
Honeycomb changes	Rare	Yes	Rare	No
Hyaline membranes	Yes, often focal	No	No	No

INTERSTITIAL LUNG DISEASES PRODUCING AN ALVEOLAR FILLING PATTERN ON CHEST RADIOGRAPH	
Alveolar proteinosis	Proteinaceous fluid
Alveolar cell carcinoma	Malignant cells
Bronchioalveolar metastases	Malignant cells from pancreas, breast
Pulmonary lymphoma	Malignant lymphocytes
Lymphocytic interstitial pneumonia	Lymphoplasmacytic cells
Alveolar sarcoid	Lymphocyte-macrophage alveolitis or confluent granuloma
Idiopathic pulmonary fibrosis-desquamative	Alveolar macrophages
Diffuse alveolar hemorrhage	Red blood cells, hemosiderin-filled macrophages
Eosinophilic pneumonia	Eosinophils, macrophages, lymphocytes
Alveolar microlithiasis	Calcium-phosphate microliths
Bronchiolitis obliterans- organizing pneumonia (BOOP)	Collagen
Mineral oil aspiration	Lipid-filled macrophages
Acute hypersensitivity pneumonia	Lymphoplasmacytic cells

IMAGING FINDING

For better understanding and diagnosis of lung disease, the pathogenesis involving the lung interstitium can be sub-grouped under,
1. Diseases characterized primarily by linear and reticular opacities.
2. Diseases characterized by nodular and reticular-nodular opacities
3. Diseases characterized primarily by increased density
4. Diseases characterized primarily by decreased lung opacity, including cystic abnormalities, emphysema, bronchiectasis.

Diseases Characterized Primarily by Linear and Reticular Opacities

The various pathological entities, which demonstrate linear and reticular opacities, can be sub-classified into:
1. Chronic interstitial pneumonias and idiopathic pulmonary fibrosis
2. Drug-induced lung diseases
3. Radiation pneumonitis
4. Asbestosis and asbestos related diseases

Chronic Interstitial Pneumonia and Idiopathic Pulmonary Fibrosis

In 1960, Leibon classified chronic interstitial pneumonias into five sub-groups based on their histological differences.

Usual interstitial pneumonias
Desquamative interstitial pneumonias
Lymphocytic interstitial pneumonias
Giant cell interstitial pneumonias
Bronchiolitis with interstitial pneumonias

The two most common presentations are UIP and DIP.

Lymphocytic interstitial pneumonia, a rare presentation of chronic interstitial pneumonia is now considered to be a pre-lymphomatous condition, except in patients with AIDS. This is a result of presence of mature lymphocytic and plasma cell infiltrates.

Usual Interstitial Pneumonias and Desquamative Interstitial Pneumonias

UIP and DIP are representations or reactions of lung to disease pathology. They are not a distinct disease process and represent different phases or stage of abnormalities caused by lung injury or disease state.

Usual interstitial pneumonias. This is the more common variety and is characterized histologically by alveolitis and increased cellularity of alveolar wall. As the process progresses, fibrosis and honeycombing develops. The end stage of UIP is idiopathic pulmonary fibrosis/cryptogenic fibrosing alveolitis. However, the latter terminology is reserved for specific pathologies leading to UIP, namely, collagen vascular diseases such as rheumatoid arthritis and scleroderma or certain drug reactions. On HRCT, UIP is characterized by a predominance of reticular opacities, which correspond to areas of irregular fibrosis, lung destruction, honeycombing and traction bronchiectasis. These findings show a peripheral sub-pleural and basal predominance. Ground-glass opacity is seen in less than 50% of cases.

Desquamative Interstitial Pneumonias is characterized by mild symptoms, mild fibrosis and large number of cells in alveolar airspaces, which represent macrophages. On HRCT the spectrum of abnormalities is similar to UIP, however fibrosis is seen in a milder form (upto 50%) and ground-glass opacity in a more extensive manner, involving all the patients with DIP. Like UIP, DIP is predominantly seen in the sub-pleural peripheral lung and in basal segments.

Idiopathic Pulmonary Fibrosis

Idiopathic pulmonary fibrosis or cryptogenic fibrosing alveolitis is seen in patients aged 40 to 60 years. As the name suggests, the cause is unknown. Pathologically, the spectrum of disease extends from that seen in UIP to DIP. Thus the finding shown in individual cases range from those typically of alveolitis with many intra-alveolar mononuclear cells and little fibrosis (DIP) to those of extensive fibrosis with relatively few intra-alveolar cells (UIP).

Findings of both UIP and DIP can be seen in same patients pointing to the fact that they can be spectrum of same disease with UIP being more severe. On HRCT the hallmark of IPF is presence of reticular opacities. The predominant HRCT findings include:
1. Findings of fibrosis as evident by intralobular interstitial thickening, irregular interfaces between the lung, vessels, bronchi, visible intralobular bronchioles, subpleural lines, honeycombing and traction bronchiectasis.
2. Irregular interlobular septal thickening which is less conspicuous than intralobular septal thickening and honeycombing.
3. Ground-glass opacity suggestive of disease activity and potentially treatable disease, however in association with fibrosis, inactivity is suggested.
4. Peripheral and subpleural predominance of abnormalities
5. Lower lung zone and posterior predominance.

Collagen Vascular Disease

Most collagen vascular diseases can cause chronic interstitial pneumonias with clinical, radiological, pathological and HRCT features indistinguishable from those of IPF. Other features commonly seen in collagen vascular diseases include pleural effusion and pleural thickening. Among the collagen vascular diseases that involve the lung, rheumatoid arthritis and scleroderma are the commonest.

Rheumatoid Arthritis: Is commonly associated with thoracic abnormalities include interstitial pneumonia and fibrosis, pleural effusion or pleural thickening, necrobiotic nodules, bronchiectasis and bronchiolitis obliterans.

Upto 90% of patients with pulmonary manifestation of RA have preceding joint disease and high Rheumatoid Factors. The HRCT findings are indistinguishable from IPF. In background of IPF additional findings may include nodules 3 mm to 3 cm (22%), consolidation (6%), lymph node enlargement (9%), pleural effusion and thickening (16%).

Progressive Systemic Sclerosis or Scleroderma

Upto 75% of patients with PSS have positive HRCT findings but only 1% shows symptoms of pulmonary dysfunction.

The HRCT findings are indistinguishable from IPF however, sub-pleural lines, parenchymal bands and honeycombing which all show a lower lung predominance are more common. Other findings include diffuse pleural thickening, asymptomatic esophageal dilatation (40-80%) and enlarged mediastinal nodes.

Mixed Connective Tissue Diseases

This entity is associated with clinical and laboratory findings overlapping those of PSS, SLE and polymyositis-dermatomyositis. The HRCT findings are similar to IPF. Additional findings include pleural effusion and pleural thickening. Pulmonary vasculitis with pulmonary hypertension and pulmonary hemorrhage are associated with MCTD.

Systemic Lupus Erythematosis

Common finding is that of pulmonary edema and pleural thickening (85%). The parenchymal lung disease in SLE is that of pneumonia, lupus pneumonitis and pulmonary hemorrhage, which present as ground-glass opacities. HRCT findings similar to UIP are rare.

Ankylosing Spondylitis

Lung involvement is seen in very few patients including 1% in largest study. HRCT shows apical pleural involvement with apical infiltrates which progress to cyst formation. The cavity may get secondarily infected by Aspergillosis or any other organism. Disease begins unilaterally and progresses bilaterally.

Drug Induced Lung Diseases

Many drugs can be associated with lung diseases but the highest incidence of adverse effects occurs with cytotoxic agents. Some of the commonest culprits include bleomycin, busulfan, vincristine, methotrexate, adriamycin and cremastin. Among the non-cytotoxic drugs the commonest include nitrofurantoin, amiodarone, gold and penicillamine.

The four patterns of drug related lung injury have been described. They are:
1. Chronic pneumonitis and fibrosis
2. Hypersensitivity lung disease
3. Non-cardiogenic pulmonary edema including the adult respiratory distress syndrome
4. Bronchiolitis obliterans

Chronic pneumonitis and fibrosis (UIP and DIP) demonstrate signs of fibrosis that is honeycombing, intralobular interstitial thickening, irregular interfaces and traction bronchiectasis. A less common finding of ground-glass opacity is seen. The lesions are predominantly peripheral and subpleural at lower and posterior lung zones.

Hypersensitivity lung disease is demonstrated by areas of ground-glass opacity.
Pulmonary edema and bronchiolitis obliterans are less frequent and the latter is caused by pencillamine and sulfasalazine only.

Radiation Pneumonitis and Fibrosis

Many factors are associated with lung reaction to radiation. In general radiological findings of radiation pneumonitis are seldom detected with doses below 3000 cGy, variably present with doses between 3000-4000 cGy and nearly always visible at doses of 4000 cGy.

The hallmarks of early radiation pneumonitis on HRCT are patchy or dense consolidation and areas of ground-glass opacity, which are confined to the radiation port. Radiation fibrosis a sequelae of early radiation pneumonitis is apparent by streaky opacities, dense consolidation with volume loss and traction bronchiectasis largely limited to radiation port.

Asbestosis and Asbestos related Diseases

Inhalation of asbestos fibres has been known to cause pulmonary and pleural abnormalities grouped as Asbestosis, Asbestos related round atelectasis and Asbestos related pleural disease.

A. *Asbestosis:* This pathology is defined as interstitial pulmonary fibrosis associated with the presence of intra-pulmonary asbestos bodies or asbestos fibres. The fibrosis initially involves the peribronchial region and later on progresses to involve the alveolar walls, interlobular septae. In advanced cases honeycombing and visceral pleural thickening is seen.

Plain radiograph has proved to be relatively insensitive in detecting the presence of asbestosis. HRCT technique for diagnosis of asbestosis is different from the routine techniques. Scans are taken at every 2 cm in both supine and prone position. This is to differentiate the normal dependent posterior lung collapse from fibrosis.

B. On HRCT, asbestosis can result in a variety of findings, depending on the severity of the disease.

- The earliest abnormal findings include centrilobular and peribronchiolar fibrosis in the form of 'dot' like opacities seen few millimeters from the pleural surface. Later the fibrosis progresses to involve the remainder of lung giving the pattern similar to IPF.
- Parenchymal bands are a common finding and reflect thickening of septae, fibrosis along bronchovascular sheath, areas of atelectasis or coarse scar. Parenchymal bands are particularly common in patients with asbestosis.
- Subpleural lines reflect early fibrosis. In more severe cases they may reflect areas of honeycombing and atelectasis.
- Parietal pleural thickening and plaques is among the most common and most helpful HRCT features in diagnosing asbestosis.
- Ground-glass opacity is seen in patients with asbestosis and correlates with presence of mild alveolar wall and interlobular septal fibrosis or edema.
- The findings are usually bilateral somewhat symmetrical and initially involve the posterior and basal lung zones.

C. *Round atelectasis and focal fibrotic masses:* This finding is seen in up to 10% of individuals with asbestosis and refers to the presence of focal lung collapse with or without folding of lung parenchyma. In order to suggest the diagnosis of rounded atelectasis on the basis of HRCT, the opacity should be
- Round or oval in shape
- Peripheral in location and abutting the pleural surface
- Associated with curving of pulmonary vessels or bronchi into the edge of the lesion (Comet tail sign) and associated with an ipsilateral pleural abnormality either effusion or pleural thickening.

D. Asbestos related pleural disease: This can be in the form of pleural effusion, pleural thickening or pleural calcification.
- Pleural effusion can be an early manifestation of asbestosis. It can be unilateral/bilateral and symmetrical.
- Pleural thickening is a common feature. When present with lung fibrosis they are pathognomic of asbestosis. The predominating sites include posterolateral costal pleural surfaces and along the surface of diaphragm. Pleural thickening is readily recognized as smooth and sharply defined thickening of pleura more than 1-2 mm from the extra pleural fat. Pleural calcification is seen in 10-20% of patients with pleural thickening. Paravertebral pleural thickening and mediastinal pleural thickening are seen in 40% of patients with asbestosis. Diffuse pleural thickening is another less common presentation of asbestosis. It is associated with pleural thickening of at least 5 cm in lateral dimensions and 8 cm in craniocaudal dimension.

DISEASES CHARACTERIZED PRIMARILY BY NODULAR AND RETICULONODULAR OPACITY

This group of lung diseases can be sub-grouped into:
1. Neoplastic lesions
   - Lymphangitis carcinomatosis
   - Hematogenous metastasis
   - Bronchioalveolar carcinoma
   - Kaposi's sarcoma
2. Granulomatous diseases
   - Sarcoidosis
3. Inhalation diseases
   - Silicosis
   - Pneumoconiosis
4. Infections
   - Mycobacterial organism
   - Fungal organisms

Neoplastic Lesions

a) Pulmonary lymphangitic carcinomatosis:
This term refers to tumor growth in the lymphatic system of the lungs. It occurs most commonly in patients with carcinoma of breast, lung, stomach, pancreas, prostate, cervix, thyroid and in patients with metastatic adenocarcinoma from an unknown primary. Pulmonary lymphangitic carcinomatosis usually results from hematogenous spread to lung, with subsequent interstitial and lymphatic invasion and from direct lymphatic spread of tumor from mediastinal and hilar lymph nodes.

The radiographic manifestations of pulmonary lymphangitis carcinomatosa includes perihilar reticular opacities, septal lines, hilar and mediastinal lymphadenopathy and pleural effusion.

HRCT findings include:

- Thickening of peribronchovascular interstitium surrounding the vessels and bronchi at the perihilar lung also called "peribronchial cuffing". This can be diffuse, local or asymmetric. The thickened peribronchovascular interstitium may be smooth and concentric or it can be nodular, a finding highly pathognomic of pulmonary lymphangitis carcinomatosis. In both instances the thickened interstitium shows a sharp interface with the adjacent aerated lung.
- Interlobular septal thickening and subpleural interstitial thickening that can be smooth or nodular and beaded. This pattern is most pronounced in periphery of the lung, so called peripheral lines or peripheral arcades. The thickened septae can be of 1-2 cm in length. A typical pattern of interlobular septal thickening that outlines a distinct pulmonary lobule is termed "polygonal arcade" seen in approximately 50% of patients. The arcades demonstrate a visible central branching opacity or dot corresponding to the thickened interstitium surrounding the interlobular artery and bronchi.
- Smooth or nodular thickening of fissure is a finding seen due to subpleural interstitial thickening, which is accentuated by the double layer in the fissural sites.
- Lymph node enlargement and pleural effusion is a less common finding seen in up to 50% of patients. Common groups involved include bronchopulmonary, tracheobronchial and mediastinal group of lymph nodes. It is important to note that PLC does not alter the lung architecture and the intervening lung parenchyma maintains its normal appearance.

b) *Hematogenous metastasis:*

In many patients hematogenous tumor metastasis to the lung results in the presence of localized tumor nodules rather that interstitial invasion. On plain radiograph multiple large well-defined nodules, randomly distributed in lung fields can be seen.

HRCT typically shows multiple small discrete nodules that have peripheral and basal appearance when limited and random distribution when innumerable. The nodules are not related to any lobule or segment, however at times they are visible in relation to vessels or pleural surfaces.

c) *Bronchioalveolar carcinoma:*

BAC can be present as solitary nodules or mass in 43% of patients, as an area of focal or diffuse consolidation in 30% and/or as a diffuse abnormality characterized by ill-defined nodules in 27% of patients. Solitary nodules will have a typical spiculated appearance. Areas of consolidation associated with BAC represent the presence of intra-alveolar tumor growth accumulation of mucin and fluid produced by the tumor. This finding is demonstrated on HRCT as patchy areas of consolidation that are peribronchovascular and contain air-bronchograms or air filled cystic spaces or extensive centrilobular air space nodules. Another possible HRCT presentation of BAC is diffuse small nodules mimicking the appearance of hematogenous metastasis. On contrast study the intratumoral vessels enhance giving the "CT angiogram sign".

d) *Kaposi's sarcoma:*

Seen approximately in 20% of patients with AIDS and pulmonary involvement occurs in 15% of these patients. HRCT findings of Kaposi's sarcoma include:

- Irregular, ill-defined peribronchovascular nodules which at times are called flame shaped nodules.
- Peribronchovascular interstitial thickening
- Pleural effusion
- Lymphadenopathy, interlobular septal thickening and ground-glass opacity are among the less common features seen in up to 1/3rd of cases.

2. Granulomatous diseases:

a. Sarcoidosis: This is a systemic disorder of unknown etiology characterized by the presence, in all of several affected organs and tissues of non-caseating epithelioid cell granulomas, proceeding either to resolution or to conversion into featureless hyaline connective tissue. The most common mode of presentation is with erythema nodosa. The sarcoidosis can be confirmed by positive Kviem test or by biopsy evidence of widespread noncaseating granulomas in more than one organ. Pulmonary manifestations are seen in up to 90% of patients. Sarcoidosis may be staged according to the appearance of chest radiograph. Stage I showing lymphadenopathy, Stage II showing lymphadenopathy with parenchymal opacities and Stage III showing parenchymal opacities alone.

HRCT findings of sarcoidosis include:

- Small, well-defined nodules seen in relation to peribronchovascular regions, adjacent to parahilar vessels and bronchi, adjacent to major fissures and in the costal subpleural regions. The nodules can be scanty or numerous and usually show an upper lobe predominance.
- Sarcoid granulomas usually cause nodular thickening of the parahilar and peribronchovascular interstitium in the form of peribronchovascular cuffing and centrilobular nodules, interlobular septae and costal subpleural region (at times termed 'pseudoplaques').
- Confluence of granulomas may result in large opacities with ill-defined contours or areas of frank consolidation. These large nodules show upper lobe predominance, airbronchograms and rarely may cavitate.
- Ground-glass opacity is seen in some patients with sarcoidosis and represent areas of disease activity.
- As the disease progresses areas of fibrosis tend to be more evident. This may be a feature of healing or progression of the disease. The most common early fibrotic changes are seen as posterior displacement of the main and upper lobe bronchi due to volume loss in the posterior segment of upper lobe. As a pathognomic feature traction bronchiectasis is seen in more advanced cases of sarcoidosis. Honeycombing is infrequent and a late feature of sarcoidosis.
- Hilar and paratracheal lymphadenopathy is an early feature of sarcoidosis. Lymphadenopathy can present with or without parenchymal changes and as the disease progresses it usually disappears within 6-12 months. Lymphadenopathy is asymmetrical and usually right-sided. A minority of nodes ultimately calcify, sometimes in characteristic eggshell fashion.

3. Inhalation Disorders

Silicosis and coal workers' pneumoconiosis are distinct diseases with differing histology and causative factors however the radiographic and HRCT appearances are quite similar and they cannot be easily or reliably distinguished.[51]

Silicosis is caused by inhalation of crystallized silicon dioxide, seen in association with heavy metal mining and hard rock mining. Pathologically the lung lesions are centrilobular and peribronchial nodules consisting of layers of laminated connective tissue. Focal emphysema surrounding the nodules are common and the nodules are seen predominantly in the upper zones.

Coal workers' pneumoconiosis results from inhalation of coal dust. It is characterized pathologically by coal macules which are accumulation of coal dust surrounded by a small amount of fibrous tissue, however the amount of fibrosis is much less than silicosis. Coal macules are also surrounded by focal areas of emphysema.

In both silicosis and coal workers' pneumoconiosis the advanced disease shows large areas of opacity or conglomerate masses. These areas exceed 1 cm and are seen in upper lobe and grows towards the hilum.

Hilar lymphadenopathy is seen in both conditions, however eggshell calcification of lymph node is pathognomic of silicosis. If present in CWP it suggests presence of silica in coal dust.

The characteristic HRCT findings include:

- Multiple nodules of 2-5 mm in size seen in peribronchial or subpleural areas. The nodules appear to be more well defined in silicosis. Nodules are seen diffusely and bilaterally and show an upper lobe and posterior predominance.
- Conglomerate mass or progressive massive fibrosis is seen in advanced cases. In CWP the mass is oval in shape, seen in background of small nodules, can be associated with areas of calcification and if larger than 4 cm will show areas of necrosis. In silicosis the mass like lesion is associated with areas of scarring and adjacent bullous changes (irregular or cicatricial emphysema).
- Hilar lymphadenopathy is seen in up to 38% of patients and eggshell calcification is pathognomic of silicosis.

4. Infection

a) Tuberculosis:

A mycobacterial infection, it has been traditionally considered in two stages, primary infection and reactivation or post-primary infection. In fact in individual cases a clear distinction between these two types of disease may be impossible.

Primary pulmonary tuberculosis is acquired by the inhalation of air-borne organism. The initial site of infection is variable but the middle and lower lung zones are first involved.

A focal pneumonitis typically results with subsequent caseous necrosis and lymphatic spread of organism to hilar and mediastinal lymph nodes. In 90-95% of patient's immunity develops leading to parenchymal and hilar granulomas. Radiographically, these patients demonstrate consolidation (50% of patients) involving the middle and lower lobes, hilar lymphadenopathy (35%), cavitation and segmental atelectasis. In 5-10% of patients, the primary tuberculosis is not resolved due to poor immunity and it leads to progressive primary tuberculosis which demonstrated in the form of extensive cavitation of the tuberculous pneumonia.

With the development of delayed hypersensitivity, pulmonary granulomas heal with fibrosis. Reactivation of postprimary tuberculosis can be seen in these individuals mainly in the upper lobe (up to 90%).

Radiographically this is demonstrated as patchy consolidation or streaky opacities (100%) seen primarily in the apical and posterior segments of upper lobes (91%), cavitatory lesions in up to 45% of patients and less commonly bronchogenic spread of disease with ill-defined nodules, fibrosis and pleural effusion.

HRCT findings seen in tuberculosis are numerous and varied and reflect the protean manifestation of this disease. These include:

- Patchy infiltration or bilateral air space consolidation usually confined to a segment and frequently peribronchial in distribution. These lesions may undergo cavitation which are usually thick walled.
- Findings suggestive of endobronchial spread of infection manifesting itself as poorly defined nodules or rosettes of nodules, 2-10 mm in diameter which can often be identified as centrilobular and/or branching centrilobular opacities appropriately described as "tree-in-bud" appearance. It is important to diagnose manifestations of endobronchial spread of tuberculosis as it denotes early course of the disease, which can be treated effectively.
- Miliary tuberculosis results in very fine, nodular or reticulonodular pattern, with nodules evenly distributed throughout the lung. The nodules measure up to 3 mm in size involving intralobular, interlobular, subpleural and perivascular interstitium.
- Hilar and mediastinal lymph nodes are seen on HRCT in patients with active disease. Right paratracheal and tracheobronchial nodes predominate. Lymph nodes larger than 2 cm show central areas of caseating necrosis.
- Pleural abnormalities in tuberculosis include pleural effusion that can be associated with pleural thickening.

b) Non-tubercular mycobacterial infections:

A number of species of non-tubercular mycobacteria have been identified but pulmonary disease is usually a result of *Mycobacterium kansasii* or organisms classified as belonging to *Mycobacterium avium intercellulare* complex.

The HRCT/CT findings of classical non-tuberculous mycobacterium mimics that of tuberculosis. The non-classical manifestations are caused by *Mycobacterium avium intercellulare* complex (MAC). These patients have propensity for areas of bronchiectasis (80%), consolidation and ground-glass opacity (73%), nodules (70%) and evidence of scarring or volume loss in 28% of cases.

c) Fungal diseases:

Fungal infection of lung has taken on a new significance after the advent of HIV infection and AIDS. Some of the more common fungal infections include histoplasmosis (histoplasma capsulatum), cryptococcosis (*Cryptococcus neoformans*), coccidioidomycosis (coccidioides immitis) and aspergillus infection (*Aspergillus fumigatus*).

Except for invasive pulmonary aspergillosis in immunocompromized patients HRCT manifestations of fungal infection cannot be differentiated from one another and are indistinguishable from those described for mycobacteria infection.

HRCT findings include both focal and diffuse parenchymal infiltrates, cavitation, nodules, hilar and mediastinal adenopathy and pleural disease. In general the accurate diagnosis of a fungal infection requires confirmation by histological examination or culture.

Invasive pulmonary aspergillosis commonly results in scattered foci of pulmonary parenchymal inflammation, infarcts and necrosis which reflect hematogenous dissemination of the fungal organisms associated with vascular obstruction. An important finding on HRCT is lower attenuation opacity surrounding the focal dense parenchymal nodules termed as "halo sign". When this sign is present in the background of HIV infection the possibility of invasive aspergillosis is to be considered.

DISEASES CHARACTERISED PRIMARILY BY INCREASED PARENCHYMAL OPACIFICATION

This group of disorders causing parenchymal opacification can be sub-grouped based on their primary manifestation as ground-glass opacity, consolidation, and parenchymal opacifications ranging from ground-glass opacity to consolidation.

Ground-glass opacity is the main abnormality seen in patients with hypersensitivity pneumonitis (extrinsic allergic alveolitis), desquamative interstitial pneumonia, and alveolar proteinosis and in diffuse pneumonias such as *Pneumocystis carinii* pneumonia.

Parenchyma consolidation is seen most commonly in bronchiolitis obliterans organizing pneumonias (BOOP), chronic eosinophilic pneumonias and bacterial pneumonias.

Parenchymal opacifications ranging between ground-glass opacity and consolidation may be seen in pulmonary edema, ARDS, viral, tubercular or fungal pneumonias, radiation pneumonitis and infarctions.

Hypersensitivity Pneumonitis (Extrinsic Allergic Alveolitis)

This entity is an allergic lung disease caused by the inhalation of antigens contained in variety of organic dusts. The major causes of EAA include:

Disease	Source of antigen
Farmer's lung	Mouldy hay
Bagassosis	Mouldy sugarcane
Mushroom workers' lung	Mushroom compost
Air conditioner/humidifier disease	Dust or mist
Malt workers' lung	Mouldy barley
Bird fanciers' lung	Avian protein from droppings and feathers

The radiographic and pathologic abnormalities seen in extrinsic allergic alveolitis is quite similar regardless of the antigen. These abnormalities can be classified into acute, subacute and chronic stages.

In acute stage, there is evidence of diffuse ill-defined air space consolidation on radiograph, which reflects alveolar filling by immunity cells.

In subacute stage, following several days of the initial episode, fine nodular pattern is seen which corresponds to areas of alveolitis, interstitial infiltrates, small granulomas and cellular bronchiolitis.

The chronic stage which follows months or years after the initial episode is characterized by areas of fibrosis which resemble IPF and honeycombing on imaging.

HRCT appearance includes:

- In acute stage it shows ill-defined small rounded opacities and areas of consolidation. HRCT does not show any superiority over plain CT in this stage.
- However in subacute stage HRCT shows patchy ground-glass opacities which are usually bilateral and small ill-defined nodules, and at times nodular ground-glass opacities that are usually centrilobular in distribution, bilateral and show no zonal predilection.
- Chronic extrinsic allergic alveolitis is characterized by findings of fibrosis which show interlobular interstitial thickening, irregular interfaces, irregular interlobular septal thickening, visible intralobular bronchioles, honeycombing and traction bronciectasis. These areas of fibrosis show patchy or random distribution with relative sparing of costophrenic angles. Other findings include poorly defined, small nodular opacities and areas of ground-glass opacity seen mainly in the mid and lower zones.

Alveolar Proteinosis

Pulmonary alveolar proteinosis (PAP) is a disease characterized by filling of the alveolar spaces with a PAS positive proteinaceous material rich in lipid. The disease is seen in all age groups but most common from 30-50 years and shows a male dominance 4:1. Chest radiograph shows a bilateral patchy, diffuse or perihilar ill-defined nodular or confluent air space pattern that is most severe in lung bases. The finding closely resembles pulmonary edema except for absence of cardiomegaly and pleural effusion.

HRCT findings range from ill-defined nodular opacities (air space nodules) to large areas of confluent air space consolidation. These areas may be sharply demarcated from the surrounding normal parenchyma giving abnormal areas of geographic pattern. The areas of ground-glass opacity may show smooth septal thickening. A combination of ground-glass opacities with intervening interlobular septal thickening gives the "crazy paving" appearance, which is strongly suggestive of alveolar proteinosis.

Bronchiolitis Obliterans Organizing Pneumonia (BOOP)/Cryptogenic Organizing Pneumonia (COP)

BOOP/COP is a disease characterized pathologically by the presence of granulation polyps within the lumina of bronchioles and alveolar ducts and patchy areas of organizing pneumonia, consisting largely of mononuclear cells and foamy macrophages in the surrounding lung. These patients present with several month history of nonproductive cough, low grade fever, shortness of breath and malaise. Pulmonary function test shows restrictive pattern. Radiological features consist of patchy non-segmental unilateral or bilateral areas of air space consolidation. Occasionally irregular opacities and small nodular opacities may be seen.

HRCT demonstrates:

- Patchy consolidation (80% of cases) or ground-glass opacity (60% of cases) often with subpleural and/or peribronchial distribution.
- Less common findings include small ill-defined nodules (30-50%) which may be peribronchial or peribronchiolar and bronchial wall thickening or dilatation seen in abnormal lung areas.

Diffuse Pneumonias

Diffuse pneumonias are caused by a variety of organisms. They are most commonly seen in immuno-compromised patients including those with malignancy, AIDS and on immunosuppressant therapy. Usually there is no requirement of HRCT for diagnosis of diffuse pneumonias, as the HRCT pattern seen in this group is mainly of consolidation and shows no specific association. Plain X-ray with clinical signs and symptoms can be enough for diagnosis. HRCT however plays a role in specific presumptive diagnosis to be made in immuno-compromised patients to assess their individual response to therapy and to differentiate the findings from the non-infectious infiltrative disease. The HRCT appearances of PCP and CMV pneumonia have been notably established.

Pneumocystis Carinii Pneumonia (PCP)

PCP affects approximately 65% of all HIV infected patients at some point during course of their disease.[60] It is currently a routine practice to put the AIDS patient with CD4 + T-lymphocyte counts less than 200 cells/mm^3 on prophylactic aerosolized pentamidine and/or trimethoprim-sulphamethoxazole combination. A definitive diagnosis of PCP requires demonstration of organism in sputum or bronchial lavage.

Radiologically and pathologically PCP is typically associated with foaming intra-alveolar exudates which appear as medium reticular or nodular opacities or areas of ill-defined hazy consolidation, which are usually perihilar. Atypical patterns of distribution are not unusual and it may demonstrate areas of cavitation, vascular invasion, vasculitis and even non-caseating calcified granulomas. This presents as asymmetric and/or nodular infiltrates, apical disease, cavitatory nodules, cysts, miliary nodules, adenopathy, effusion and pneumothoraces. Of particular interest is development of cysts and pneumothorax, which is seen in up to 10% of cases and measures up to 5 cm in diameter.

HRCT findings

- The most common finding includes areas of ground-glass opacity and/or consolidation, which show central and perihilar predilection. In addition to this diffuse pattern, a distinct mosaic pattern could be identified with areas of normal lung scattered in between the involved parenchyma. In up to 50% of patients thickened septal lines are seen in association with areas of ground-glass opacities. Kuhlman *et al* found this patterns of HRCT involvement, including ground-glass opacity, patch work pattern and interstitial or reticular pattern.
- Atypical manifestations of PCP include cystic abnormalities 38%, nodular densities 18%, adenopathy 18% and effusion 18%. The cysts seen in PCP follow a predictable evolution. Initially, cysts appear as small foci in areas of consolidation, often associated with clearly dilated thick walled bronchi. With time these cysts coalesce to form bizarre shaped, thick walled cysts that often appear septated. There is a high tendency for sub-pleural cysts to communicate with the pleura, accounting for pneumothorax.
- PCP findings can reflect the stage of the disease. In acute stage there is evidence of scattered foci of ground-glass opacity or air space consolidation can be identified with some degree of alveolar thickening. In treated

patients with resolving or subacute infection, reticular opacities representing thickened interlobular septa and intralobular lines can be seen in association with ground-glass opacities. In chronic cases, following therapy the residual changes usually include areas of bronchiectasis and fibrosis.

Cytomegalovirus (CMV) Pneumonia

CMV frequently occurs in immunosuppressed patients specially following organ transplantation. The chest X-ray findings in recipients with pulmonary infiltrates shows CMV with an incidence of up to 90% in patients with bone marrow transplantation when compared to PCP (4%) and other bacterial or yeast infections (6%). CMV is well recognized as the most common viral organism to be identified in patients with AIDS.

HRCT shows patchy bilateral foci of ground-glass opacification and/or consolidation, which may resemble that of early PCP. Less common features include multiple, scattered poorly defined nodules and bilateral reticular changes.

Acute Interstitial Pneumonia (AIP)

AIP is a fulminant disease of unknown etiology that usually occurs in a previously healthy person and produces histological findings of diffuse alveolar damage. The pathological abnormalities consist of thickening of the alveolar walls due to edema, inflammatory cells and active fibroblast proliferation but little mature collagen deposition. This entity is clinically and pathologically distinct from UIP and DIP. Because the acute presentation and the histologic features are identical with those of ARDS, AIP is also been referred to as idiopathic ARDS.

Radiograph is characterized by bilateral air space opacification involving mainly the upper zones.

Honeycombing is seen only in a few percentage of patients.

HRCT demonstrates bilateral symmetrical areas of ground-glass opacity involving all lung zones equally. Less commonly areas of air space consolidation and subpleural honeycombing is seen.

DISEASES CHARACTERIZED PRIMARILY BY DECREASED LUNG OPACITY, INCLUDING CYSTIC ABNORMALITIES, EMPHYSEMA AND BRONCHIECTASIS

Many groups of diseases have in common the presence of focal, multifocal or diffuse decrease in lung opacity. These diseases include pulmonary histocytosis X, lymphangiomyomatosis, different types of emphysema and airway diseases including bronchiectasis and diseases primarily affecting small airways such as bronchiolitis obliterans and panbronchiolitis.

Pulmonary Histiocytosis X

Pulmonary histiocytosis X is an idiopathic disease characterized in its early stages by granulomatous nodules containing Langerhan's histiocytes and eosinophils, which are primarily peribronchial in distribution. The disease is seen in young and middle aged adults showing male dominance and up to 90% of patients giving history of smoking. Radiographic finding consists of reticular, nodular, reticulonodular patterns and honeycombing often in combination.

HRCT findings demonstrate:
- Multiple cysts which are usually less than 10 mm in diameter however larger cysts can occur. The cysts can be thin walled (< 2 mm) or thick walled (> 2 mm) the former being more common. Majority of the cysts are round, however they can also have bizarre shapes, being bilobed, cloverleaf shaped or branching in appearance. These cysts show an upper lobe predominance.

- In majority of cases associated nodules are seen measuring less than 5 mm. Larger nodules are rare and there may be areas of cavitation. The margins of the nodules are irregular and are seen to be peribronchial or peribronchiolar.
- Cysts and nodules show upper lobe predominance with sparing of costophrenic angles.

Lymphangiomyomatosis

This is a rare disease characterized by progressive proliferation of spindle cells, resembling immature smooth muscles, in the lung parenchyma and along lymphatic vessels in chest and abdomen. Proliferation of spindle cells along the bronchioles leads to air trapping and the development of emphysema and thin walled lung cysts. The disease exclusively involves women of childbearing age. The plain radiograph manifestation of lymphangiomyomatosis includes reticular, reticulonodular and honeycombing pattern. Associated pleural effusion and pneumothorax is commonly seen.

HRCT demonstrates:
- Lung cysts which are usually 2-5 mm in diameter but can be larger. They are thin walled and distributed randomly throughout the lung.
- Hilar and mediastinal lymph node is seen in up to 50% of patients.
- Less common findings include linear interstitial markings, interlobular septal thickening or patchy areas of ground-glass opacity.

Emphysema

Emphysema is defined as a condition of lung characterized by permanent, abnormal enlargement of air spaces distal to the terminal bronchiole, accompanied by destruction of their walls. Unlike the previous belief areas of fibrosis may be present. Emphysema is usually classified into three main subtypes based on the anatomic distribution of the areas of lung destruction. The subtypes are:
- Proximal acinar, centriacinar or centrilobular emphysema
- Panacinar or panlobular emphysema
- Distal acinar or paraseptal emphysema

Centrilobular emphysema usually results from cigarette smoking and involves the upper zones. The emphysema predominantly affects the respiratory bronchioles in the central portion of acini and therefore involves the central portion of the lobules.

Panlobular emphysema is classically associated with alpha-1 antitrypsin deficiency, although it may also be seen in smokers, in the elderly and distal to bronchial and bronchiolar obliterations. Panlobular emphysema involves all the components of the acinus more or less uniformly and therefore involves the entire lobule.

Paraseptal emphysema can be an isolated phenomenon, often associated with pneumothorax or can be seen in older patients with centrilobular emphysema. Paraseptal emphysema predominantly involves the alveolar ducts and sacs, with areas of destruction often marginated by the interlobular septa.

Bullae can develop in association with any type of emphysema but are most common with paraseptal or centrilobular emphysema. It is characterized by sharply demarcated areas of emphysema measuring 1 cm or more and possessing a wall less than 1 mm in thickness. Bullae have been classified by Reid according to the location and the type of emphysema with which they are associated. According to this classification, type I bullae are subpleural in location and occur in patients with paraseptal emphysema, type II bullae are also subpleural but are associated with generalized emphysema (centrilobular/panlobular), type III bullae are associated with generalized emphysema but occur within the lung parenchyma rather than in subpleural location.

Paracicatrial or irregular emphysema is referred to as irregular air space enlargement seen in patients with pulmonary fibrosis.

HRCT findings include:
- Areas of decreased opacity (lung destruction) with or without visible walls.
- Centrilobular emphysema of mild to moderate is characterized by presence of multiple, small round areas of abnormally low attenuation, several mm in diameter distributed throughout the lung but having upper lobe predominance which lack recognizable walls. Areas of lucency are seen grouped near the centre of secondary pulmonary lobules surrounding the centrilobular artery branches. Some areas of fibrosis may be present. With more severe centrilobular emphysema the destruction can become confluent and the term confluent centrilobular emphysema is used. This appearance closely resembles panlobular emphysema.
- Panlobular emphysema is characterized by uniform destruction of the pulmonary lobule leading to widespread areas of abnormally low attenuation and it is more severe in lower lobes. Pulmonary vessels in the affected lung appear fewer and smaller than normal. At times it is difficult to detect mild to moderate areas of panlobular emphysema.
- Paraseptal emphysema is characterized by involvement of distal part of the secondary lobule and is therefore most striking in a subpleural location. Areas of subpleural, paraseptal emphysema, often have visible walls, but the walls are very thin. Usually some areas of fibrosis are also detected. When larger than 1 cm in diameter the areas of subpleural emphysema are termed as bullae. However bullae can be seen with other types of emphysema as well and they are common causes of spontaneous pneumothorax.
- Bullous emphysema reffers to the presence of emphysema associated with large bullae and is usually seen in patients with paraseptal or centrilobular emphysema. A syndrome of "bullous emphysema" or "giant bullous emphysema" has been described and is also known as "vanishing lung syndrome", "type I bullous disease" or "primary bullous disease". It is seen in young men and is characterized by the presence of large progressive upper lobe bullae, which occupy a significant volume of hemithorax (up to 1/3rd of hemithorax).
- Irregular air space enlargement also known as cicatricial emphysema is a localized area of air space enlargement found adjacent to parenchymal scars, diffuse pulmonary fibrosis and in pneumoconiosis.

Bronchiectasis

Bronchiectasis is defined as localized, irreversible dilatation of the bronchial tree. A wide variety of disorders are associated with bronchiectasis. Some of the more common conditions include infections (bacterial, mycobacterial, fungal, viral), bronchial obstruction, emphysema (Alpha-1-antitrypsin deficiency), asthma, allergic bronchopulmonary aspergillosis, cystic fibrosis, Kartagener's syndrome, immunodeficiency states, Marfan's syndrome, bronchiolitis obliterans and chronic fibrosis. In general clinical diagnosis of bronchiectasis is possible only in the most severely affected patients, and even in this setting, differentiation from chronic bronchitis may be problematic. Presenting features may include purulent sputum production, hemoptysis and recurrent respiratory infection. The radiographic manifestations of bronchiectasis have been well described. These include loss of definition of vascular markings in specific lung segments (secondary to peribronchial fibrosis and volume loss), evidence of bronchial wall thickening and in more severely affected cases the presence of discrete cystic masses occasionally containing air fluid levels. Bronchographic findings traditionally believed to be the gold standard has been called into question and include proximal and/or distal bronchial dilatation, pruning or lack of normal tapering of peripheral airways and luminal filling defects.

HRCT findings in typical cases of bronchiectasis include:

- *Bronchial dilatation:* Up to date no absolute CT criteria of normal bronchial diameter have been determined, however generally bronchiectasis is considered to be present when the internal diameter of a bronchus is greater than the diameter of the adjacent pulmonary artery. This finding is demonstrated on axial sections through bronchus as "signet ring sign". As shown by Lynch et al dilated bronchi alone cannot be associated, as a sign of bronchiectasis and other associated signs should be present as well.

- *Bronchial wall thickening:* As with bronchial diameter, there are no objective CT criteria as to normal bronchial wall thickness and this observation is also largely subjective. To diagnose bronchial wall thickening, comparison with adjacent normal bronchi is important. Also normal bronchi are visible up to the middle 1/3rd of lung and smallest airways seen are of the diameter of 2 mm with thickness of 0.2-0.3 mm. Visualization of bronchi in peripheral 2 cm of lung is suggestive of bronchial wall thickening.

- Lack of bronchial wall tapering and contour irregularities. Traditionally bronchiectasis has been classified into cylindrical, varicose and cystic varieties depending on the severity of bronchial dilatation.
  Cylindrical bronchiectasis: Mild or cylindrical bronchiectasis is diagnosed if the dilated bronchi are relatively uniform caliber and have roughly parallel walls. Depending of whether the bronchi have a horizontal or vertical course they give "tram track sign" or "signet ring appearance" respectively.
  Varicose bronchiectasis: With increasing severity of bronchiectasis, the abnormal bronchi develop a beaded configuration. This variety can be diagnosed only if the bronchi are horizontal to the beam. At times the diagnosis becomes difficult due to mucoid impaction of the bronchi.
  Cystic bronchiectasis: With severe or cystic bronchiectasis the involved airways are cystic or saccular in appearance and may extend to the pleural surface. The cysts are usually thick walled but may appear thin walled. Cystic bronchiectasis may be associated with the presence of:

- Air-fluid levels caused by retained secretions in the dependent portion of the dilated bronchi
- A string of cysts caused by sectioning irregularly dilated bronchi along the length
- Cluster of cysts
- Mucous or fluid retention in bronchial lumen. The appearance of fluid or mucus filled airways is dependent both on their size and orientation relative to CT scan plane. Fluid filled airway result in abnormal lobular or branching structures when they lie in the same plane as CT scan (tree-in-bud appearance).

A few conditions associated with bronchiectasis have been reported to have distinctive HRCT appearances that can aid in diagnosis. These include bronchiectasis in cystic fibrosis, allergic bronchopulmonary aspergillosis and non-tubercular mycobacterial infection.

Cystic fibrosis: Cystic fibrosis is the most common cause of pulmonary insufficiency in the 1st decade of life. It is an autosomal recessive disease with the defect in "cystic fibrosis transmembrane regulation protein" which leads to chloride transport across membranes. This leads to chloride transport across membranes. This leads to abnormal mucous clearance, mucous plugging of airways and an increased incidence of bacterial airway infection. This in turn leads to bronchiectasis.

HRCT findings include:

- Bronchiectasis is present in almost in all the patients and is usually perihilar, referred to as "central bronchiectasis", however in upto 2/3 of patients peripheral bronchi can be involved as well. All lobes are involved however early in the disease upper lobe is the most prominent site. Cylindrical bronchiectasis is seen in up to 94% of cases and later in the course of the disease cystic bronchiectasis is a prominent feature.
- Bronchial wall thickening and peribronchial interstitial thickening is a prominent early feature of this disease.

- Mucous plugging is also common. Branching and nodular centrilobular opacities, which reflect the presence of bronchiolar dilatation with associated mucous impaction, infection or peribronchial inflammation can be early sign of the disease.
- Less common findings includes collapse, consolidation, mediastinal lymph node enlargement and pleural abnormalities.

Allergic Bronchopulmonary Aspergillosis

This is characteristically associated with eosinophilia, symptoms of asthma such as wheezing, and findings of central or proximal bronchiectasis, mucoid impaction, atelectasis and sometimes consolidation.

HRCT findings
- Bronchiectasis is seen which is usually central and cystic in variety
- Mucoid impaction is common finding. Small airway abnormalities with dilatation of mucous or fluid filled centrilobular bronchioles, can also be seen on HRCT, resulting in tree-in-bud appearance.
- Less common findings of consolidation and segmental or subsegmental atelectasis may be seen.

Useful HRCT Patterns in the Diagnosis of Interstitial Lung Disease	
Finding	*Common Diagnoses*
By type of radiographic abnormality	
Reticular lines, honeycombing	CVD-related, IPF, asbestosis, sarcoidosis, chronic HP
Airspace opacity, "ground-glass", consolidation	BOOP, chronic EP, PAP, lymphoma, sarcoidosis
Nodules	Granulomatous diseases, pneumoconioses, malignancy
Septal thickening	Infection, edema, malignancy, drug reaction, pulmonary veno-occlusive disease, acute EP
Cystic changes	PEG, LAM
By anatomic distribution of abnormality	
Mid-upper lung zone	Hypersensitivity pneumonitis, sarcoidosis, PEG, chronic beryllium disease
Lower lung zone	CVD-related, IPF, asbestosis
Peripheral	BOOP, IPF, EP
Perihilar/peribronchovascular	Sarcoidosis, malignancy, LIP
BOOP—bronchiolitis obliterans organizing pneumonia; CVD—collagen vascular disease; EP—eosinophilic pneumonia; HP—hypersensitivity pneumonitis; IPF—idiopathic pulmonary fibrosis; LAM—lymphangioleiomyomatosis; LIP—lymphocytic interstitial pneumonitis; PAP—pulmonary alveolar proteinosis; PEG—eosinophilic	

- *Fever:* Infections (including immunodeficiency), eosinophilic pneumonia, drug reactions, vasculitis, connective tissue disorders, cryptogenic organising pneumonia, extrinsic alveolitis, sarcoidosis, AIDS, lymphoma and lymphangitic carcinoma
- *Rash:* Sarcoidosis, connetive tissue disorders, vasculitis
- *Scleritis:* Sarcoidosis, connective tissue disorders, vasculitis
- *Keratoconjunctivitis sicca:* Sjögren's syndrome
- *Uveitis:* Sarcoidosis, Behcet's syndrome, ankylosing spondylitis
- *Raynaud's phenomenon:* Systemic sclerosis, CFA

- *Systemic hypertension:* Connective tissue disorders, Goodpasture's syndrome, vasculitis
- *Lacrymal and salivary gland enlargement:* Sarcoidosis, Sjögren's syndrome
- *Lymphadenopathy:* Sarcoidosis, lymphoma, lymphangitic carcinoma, HIV
- *Pericarditis:* Connective tissue disorders, lymphangitis, lymphoma, vasculitis
- *Hepatosplenomegaly:* Sarcoidosis, LCH, connective tissue disorders, amyloidosis
- *Arthritis:* Connective tissue disorders, vasculitis, sarcoidosis, Goodpasture's syndrome
- *Haematuria:* Vasculitis
- *Oral candidiasis:* Immunodeficiency (especially HIV).

GUIDELINES TO EVALUATE DIFFUSE LUNG DISEASES

Clinical

An accurate detailed history is vital. There should be particular emphasis on coexisting or past systemic disease, medication, occupational and environmental exposures, travel, family, and smoking history, and the possibility of underlying immunosuppression, including HIV.

In addition to careful respiratory examination, there should be evaluation of systemic disease including fever, cardiac status, rashes, eye signs, hepatosplenomegaly, arthritis and urine dipstick.

The initial laboratory investigations should include full blood and eosinophil counts, viscosity or erythrocyte sedimentation rate (ESR), serum urea and electrolytes, creatinine, calcium, liver function tests, and autoantibodies (antinuclear and rheumatoid factors).

Depending on the clinical setting, further investigation may need to include additional autoantibodies [(antineutrophil cytoplasmic antibody (ANCA), glomerular basement membrane antibody (anti-GBM)], serum precipitins, electrocardiography and echocardiography. Previous radiographs or reports should be sought.

Imaging

Radiologists and respiratory physicians should meet regularly to jointly evaluate imaging in patients with DPLD.

In patients for whom the diagnosis is uncertain after chest radiography and clinical assessment, HRCT scanning is the next investigation of choice and should precede biopsy. HRCT scanning is valuable in detecting DPLD in patients with a normal chest radiograph.

HRCT scanning also provides prognostic information and is recommended in this disease irrespective of its diagnostic role.

HRCT scanning should be performed on appropriate equipment. At least once a week checks should be made with a phantom to ensure the equipment gives high quality images.

Wherever possible an extended interscan interval (20 mm) and a low dose technique should be used.

- The radiologist performing the HRCT scans should have expertise in the technique and recognise the strengths and limitations of the procedure. At least one radiologist in any department should have a declared interest and be trained in chest radiology and HRCT scanning.
- Consideration should be given to establishing a reference panel of radiologists with particular expertise in HRCTscanning.

Lung Function

- While most patients will have restrictive lung function, some DPLDs are associated with airflow obstruction or occur in patients with pre-existing airflow obstruction. A finding of airflow obstruction should not by itself lead to exclusion of a diagnosis of DPLD.

- The minimum lung function assessment should be spirometric values and gas transfer factor, which together give a reasonable measure of the extent of the disease. Vital capacity and gas transfer factor are the most appropriate lung function tools for disease monitoring.

DIFFUSE PARENCHYMAL LUNG DISEASE

They can be classified into:
1. Acute DPLD.
2. Episodic DPLD, all of which may present acutely.
3. Chronic DPLD due to occupational or environmental agents or drugs.
4. Chronic DPLD with evidence of systemic disease.
5. Chronic DPLD with no evidence of systemic disease.

Acute DPLD

Cause—Example
- Infection (bacterial including tuberculosis)
- Viral (e.g. chicken pox, measles)
- Fungal (e.g. invasive aspergillosis, histoplasmosis associated with immunodeficiency, e.g. *Pneumocystis* and cytomegalovirus)
- Allergy drugs (e.g. penicillin)
- Fungi (e.g. aspergillosis)
- Helminths (e.g. Toxocara)
- Toxins drugs (e.g. cytotoxics, amiodarone)
- Toxic gases, fumes (e.g. chlorine)
- Hemodynamic left venticular failure, fluid overload, renal failure, vasculitis/hemorrhage, Goodpasture's syndrome, idiopathic hemosiderosis, Behcet's syndrome, systemic lupus erythematosus, Wegener's granulomatosis, Churg-Strauss syndrome
- ARDS Trauma, septicemia
- Unknown cryptogenic organising pneumonia, cryptogenic pulmonary eosinophilia.

Episodic DPLD

- Eosinophilic pneumonia
- Vasculitides/pulmonary hemorrhage
- Churg-Strauss syndrome
- Extrinsic allergic alveolitis
- Cryptogenic organising pneumonia

Chronic DPLD Secondary to Occupational or Environmental Agents

Agent inhaled—Example
- Inorganic dusts
- Fibrogenic Asbestosis
- Silicosis
- Coal workers' pneumoconiosis
- Hard metal (cobalt)
- Aluminium lung

- Non-fibrogenic Siderosis (iron)
- Stannosis (tin)
- Baritosis (barium)
- Antimony
- Granulomatous/fibrogenic Berylliosis
- Organic dusts (extrinsic allergic alveolitis)
- Bacteria Farmers' lung (Thermoactinomycetes in mouldy hay)
- Bagassosis (Thermoactinomycetes in mouldy sugarcane)
- Fungi Suberosis (in cork workers)
- Cheese workers' lung (mouldy cheese)
- Animal protein Bird fanciers' lung (avian protein on feathers)
- Chemicals Pyrethrum extrinsic allergic alveolitis
- Isocyanates.

Drug and Toxin induced DPLD: Classification with Examples

- Antibiotics: Nitrofurantoin, sulphasalazine
- Anti-inflammatory agents: Gold, penicillamine, aspirin
- Cardiovascular agents: Amiodarone
- Chemotherapeutic agents: Bleomycin, methotrexate
- Drug induced SLE: Hydrallazine
- Illicit drugs: Heroin, methadone, talc
- Miscellaneous: Oxygen, radiation, lipoid pneumonia

Examples of Chronic DPLD with Evidence of Systemic Disease

- Connective tissue disorders
  Systemic sclerosis: Rheumatoid arthritis
  Systemic lupus erythematosus: Polymyositis
  Sjogren's syndrome: Mixed connective tissue disorders
  Ankylosing spondylitis: Behcet's disease
- Neoplastic
  Lymphoma: Lymphangitic carcinoma
  Micrometastates
- Vasculitis
  Wegener's granulomatosis Microscopic polyangiitis
  Goodpasture's syndrome
- Sarcoidosis
- Inherited disorders
  Tuberose sclerosis Neurofibromatosis
  Lipid storage disease Hermansky-Pudlak syndrome
- Other miscellaneous
  Inflammatory bowel disease HIV associated
  Post bone marrow transplantation Amyloidosis
  Cryptogenic organising pneumonia Miliary tuberculosis
  Langerhans' cell histiocytosis Pulmonary eosinophilia
  May be confined to the lung.

Examples of Chronic DPLD with no Evidence of Systemic Disease or External Agent Exposure

Cryptogenic fibrosing alveolitis Sarcoidosis
Cryptogenic organising pneumonia Langerhans' cell histiocytosis
Alveolar proteinosis Bronchocentric granulomatosis
Chronic aspiration Pulmonary veno-occlusive disease
Alveolar microlithiasis Idiopathic pulmonary hemosiderosis
Lymphangioleiomyomatosis Bronchoalveolar carcinoma
Pulmonary eosinophilia.

DEFINITIONS

Immunocompromised host: An individual with a defect (either inherited or acquired) in one or more host defense mechanisms which leads to increased risk of infection.

Opportunistic infection: An organism which does not cause disease in an immunocompetent host but is able to exploit a defect in the immunocompromised host.

Primary pathogen: An organism which can cause disease even in immunocompetent individuals.

Colonization: The presence of an organism in a tissue or organ system which is not normally present at that location. Unlike a pathogen, a colonizer does not invade host tissue or cause tissue destruction, but retains the ability to be a pathogen under appropriate circumstances.

DIAGNOSTIC TESTS FOR OPPORTUNISTIC INFECTIONS

Chest Radiograph

Sputum culture

Transtracheal aspiration

Blood cultures

Serologic tests

Bronchoscopic cultures

Bronchial washings

Bronchoalveolar lavage (BAL)

Transbronchoscopic lung biopsy

Transthoracic needle aspiration

Pulmonary Diseases Associated with Specific Immune System Defects

Cystic Fibrosis (CF): This is the most common lethal inherited birth defect. The defective gene has been recently discovered and is referred to as CFTR (cystic fibrosis transmembrane conductance regulator). In children, *Staphylococcus aureus* is the most common pathogen. However, as the disease progresses, gram-negative bacilli such as *Pseudomonas aeruginosa* become prominent.

Bronchiectasis: This refers to an abnormal dilation of bronchial walls. Although a congenital predisposition may occur, the majority of cases appear to be caused by chronic inflammation of bronchial walls, typically from infection. Childhood illnesses such as pertussis, and tuberculosis were once common causes, however, with the advent of antibiotics, bronchiectasis is becoming less common.

The abnormally dilated bronchial segments have impaired mucociliary clearance which leads to collection of mucus, colonization with bacteria, and frequent episodes of bronchitis and pneumonia .

Primary Ciliary Dyskinesia: A collection of hereditary defects which result in dysfunction of cilia. Structural defects in these hair-like projections results in impaired mucociliary clearance, leading to recurrent sinusitis, pneumonia, and bronchitis.

Impaired Humoral Immunity: The proper functioning of antibody production and complement are important aspects of humoral immunity. Therefore, any defect in this component of the immune system leads to impaired clearance of encapsulated organisms. These include *Streptococcus pneumoniae, Neisseria meningitidis*, and *Hemophilus influenzae*. Afflicted individuals are predisposed to developing recurrent sinusitis, otitis media, and pneumonia from these organisms.

The hereditary humoral defects include a variety of immunoglobulin and complement deficiencies. Acquired humoral defects are more common. These include splenectomy, sickle cell anemia, and various leukemias, which impair antibody production. Acquired complement deficiencies are most commonly associated with *systemic lupus erythematosus (SLE), hepatic failure and nephrotic syndrome.*

Impaired Cellular Immunity: Impaired T cell functioning predisposes the host to certain bacteria, fungi, viruses, and parasites. Bacterial pathogens include *M. tuberculosis, M. avium intracellulare, Listeria, Nocardia*, and *Legionella*. Viral pathogens include cytomegalovirus, and herpes viruses. Prominent fungal infections include *Cryptococcus, Coccidioides*, and *Histoplasma*. Parasitic organisms include *Pneumocystis, Toxoplasma*, and *Strongyloides*.

Common causes include immunosuppression due to malignancy, chemotherapy, prevention of transplant rejection, and as part of treatment for certain inflammatory conditions such as sarcoidosis, SLE, rheumatoid arthritis and asthma.

AIDS is now the most common cause of cellular immunodeficiency: The infections due to acquired cellular immunity defects are similar to those associated with HIV infection which will be discussed below.
- Host defense defects often promote bacterial pneumonia.
- Humoral defects result in impaired clearance of encapsulated organisms such as *S. pneumoniae, Neisseria meningitidis*, and *Haemophilus influenzae*.
- Cellular immune defects promote infection with TB, MAC, *Listeria, Nocardia, Legionella*, CMV, Herpes viruses, *Cryptococcus, Coccidioides, Histoplasma, Pneumocystis, Toxoplasma*, and *Strongyloides*.

Pulmonary Conditions and Infections Associated with AIDS		
Common	*Less common*	*Occasionally seen*
Bacterial pneumonia	*M. avium* complex	Toxoplasmosis
Pneumocystis pneumonia	Cryptococcosis	Cryptosporim
M.TB	Coccidioidomycosis	Strongyloides
Kaposi's sarcoma	Histoplasmosis	*M.kansasii*
	Cytomegalovirus	Legionella
	Nocardia	Aspergillus
	Lymphoma	Lymphoid and nonspecific Interstitial pneumonitis

INFECTIOUS PULMONARY COMPLICATIONS OF AIDS

Bacterial Infections
During the previous decade, it was widely maintained that *Pneumocystis carinii* was the most common cause of HIV-associated pneumonia

- Bacteria most commonly isolated in HIV-related pneumonia include *S. pneumoniae*, *H. influenzae*, and *S. aureus*. *S. aureus* is particularly common in intravenous drug users. Clinical features of bacterial pneumonia are similar to those of immunocompetent individuals.

Pneumocystis Carinii Pneumonia

Pneumocystis carinii pneumonia (PCP) is a significant cause of HIV-associated pneumonia and is a common cause of respiratory failure and death in the HIV population. Nearly 75% of those who have AIDS will develop PCP at some point during their disease process. Many have recurrent pneumonias.

- The chest radiograph most commonly reveals fluffy, perihilar alveolar and interstitial infiltrates.

Tuberculosis

Early in the course of HIV infection, when CD^{4+} counts are relatively normal, HIV-associated TB presents in a similar fashion to TB in HIV-negative individuals. TB radiographic features include apical infiltrates and cavitary disease.

In the late stages of HIV infection, TB may present with atypical features such as a miliary pattern or diffuse infiltrates. Cavitary disease is usually absent. Extrapulmonary disease is more common and may coexist with pulmonary involvement. Extrapulmonary TB may manifest as pleural effusions, thoracic or hilar lymphadenopathy, and may involve the gastrointestinal tract and bone marrow.

Atypical Mycobacteria

HIV infection also predisposes one to infection with other types of mycobacteria which do not normally cause disease in the immunocompetent individual. These organisms are referred to as *atypical* mycobacteria, and the most common type to infect HIV-positive subjects is *Mycobacterium avium complex* (MAC).

Fungal Pneumonias

HIV-infected individuals are at increased risk for several fungal infections. These include *Cryptococcus neoformans*, *Histoplasma capsulatum*, *Coccidioides immitis*, *Blastomyces dermatitidis*, and *Aspergillus fumigatus*. As many as 25% of all AIDS-defining infections are due to fungi.
Histoplasmosis
Blastomycosis
Coccidioidomycosis.

Viral Infections

Several viral pathogens are reported to cause pulmonary disease in immunosuppressed patients including varicella-zoster, herpes simplex, Epstein-Barr virus, and adenovirus. However, CMV (cytomegalovirus) is the only viral pathogen which commonly produces disease in association with HIV infection.

NONINFECTIOUS PULMONARY COMPLICATIONS OF AIDS

AIDS-Associated Malignancies
Chest radiograph, KS lesions may appear as nodular densities or interstitial infiltrates. The latter may be confused with opportunistic infections, such as *P. carinii.*

Non-Hodgkin's Lymphoma is the second most common AIDS-associated lymphoma. It is usually disseminated at the time of diagnosis, however, mediastinal or hilar lymphadenopathy is not as common as in those without HIV-infection.

HIV-Associated Interstitial Pneumonitis

Lymphocytic interstitial pneumonitis (LIP) is a diffuse infiltration of predominantly lymphocytes. Radiographic involvement shows a bilateral reticulonodular pattern, particularly in the lower lung fields.

Nonspecific interstitial pneumonitis may also occur with HIV. Radiograph typically reveals diffuse interstitial infiltrates.

Cytotoxic reactions: In patients treated with chemotherapeutic or cytotoxic agents, a diffuse interstitial pneumonitis can develop. Agents known to induce interstitial pneumonitis include bleomycin, cyclophosphamide, methotrexate, busulfan, and chlorambucil.

Radiation pneumonitis: An acute interstitial pneumonitis may develop 1-6 months after radiation therapy. The infiltrates are usually limited to the regions exposed to the radiation beam. This may progress to pulmonary fibrosis.

Pattern Approach to Infective Lesions

Segmental consolidation is usually due to bacterial pneumonia.

Nodules or *rounded masses* are often fungal, or occasionally Kaposi's sarcoma. *Lobar/segmental atelectasis* is sometimes due to aspergillosis or mucormycosis. These organisms invade vessels and cause thrombi resulting in airless infarcts. *Miliary lesions* can be tuberculosis, fungal infection, or hematogenous metastases.

Diffuse alveolar or interstitial disease suggests *Pneumocystis*, CMV, and occasionally Kaposi's sarcoma.

Noninfectious causes are also common and include pulmonary edema, transfusion reactions, drug toxicity, *lymphocytic interstitial pneumonitis*, radiation pneumonitis, and intra-alveolar hemorrhage.

Cavitary disease is suggestive of tuberculosis, coccidioidomycosis, and occasionally *M. kansasii.*

Pullouts

Pullout 1: Approach to Ground Glass Opacity

Ground glass opacity (GGO) is described as a "hazy increased attenuation of lung, with preservation of bronchial and vascular margins; it is caused by partial filling of air spaces, interstitial thickening, partial collapse of alveoli, normal expiration, or increased capillary blood volume."GGO is a nonspecific finding, and the differential diagnosis of the many causes of GGO can be lengthy. This approach gives a set of differentials for GGO according to the morphological pattern of involvement.

Causes of a diffuse pattern of GGO on CT scanning
- Acute rejection of lung transplantation
- Adult respiratory distress syndrome (ARDS)
- Edema
- Extrinsic allergic alveolitis
- Hemorrhage
- Infectious pneumonia

Causes of a patchy pattern of GGO on CT scanning
- Acute rejection of lung transplantation
- Adult respiratory distress syndrome
- Bronchiolitis obliterans organizing pneumonia (BOOP)
- Bronchioloalveolar cell carcinoma
- Extrinsic allergic alveolitis
- Hemorrhage
- Infectious pneumonia
- Pulmonary alveolar proteinosis

Causes of a focal pattern of GGO on CT scanning
- Bronchiolitis obliterans organizing pneumonia (BOOP)
- Bronchoalveolar lavage
- Bronchioloalveolar cell carcinoma
- Hemorrhage
- Pulmonary infection

Causes of a peripheral pattern of GGO on CT scanning
- Bronchiolitis obliterans organizing pneumonia (BOOP)
- Collagen vascular disease
- Contusion
- Desquamative interstitial pneumonitis
- Drug toxicity
- Eosinophilic pneumonia
- Fibrosis
- Sarcoidosis

Causes of a "halo" pattern of GGO on CT scanning
- Invasive pulmonary aspergillosis • Neoplasm, hemorrhagic • Post-biopsy pseudo nodule

Pullout 2: Approach to Bronchiolar CT Patterns

(A) The normal bronchiole has a diameter δ 1 mm and thin walls and is not usually visible on CT scans.

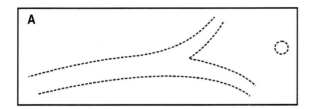

(B) When the bronchiolar wall is thickened, CT shows the abnormal bronchiole in profile or as a ring shadow in cross section in the periphery of the lung, where bronchioles are usually not seen.

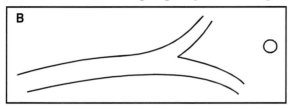

(C) Dilated bronchioles become visible on CT when they reach a diameter of ε 2 mm, the limit of visibility on CT.

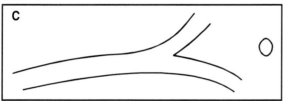

(D) Impacted bronchioles are shown as centrilobular nodular and linear branching opacities that sometimes form V shapes.

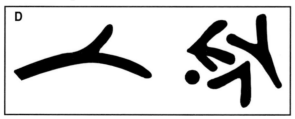

(E) The "tree-in-bud" pattern represents severe bronchiolar impaction with "clubbing" of distal bronchioles and more than one contiguous branching site.

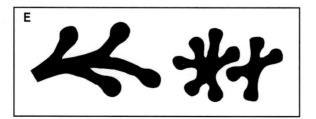

Bronchiolitis

"Bronchiolitis" is a term used to describe a spectrum of inflammatory disorders affecting small bronchioles. These disorders show great heterogeneity in regard to cause, clinical features, and histopathologic changes. Myersand Colby classified these conditions into 8 types:

1. Constrictive bronchiolitis
2. Cryptogenic organizing pneumonia
3. Infectious bronchiolitis
4. Adult bronchiolitis
5. Respiratory bronchiolitis
6. Mineral dust airways disease
7. Diffuse panbronchiolitis and
8. Follicular bronchiolitis.

Infection

Endobronchial spread of infectious organisms can result in centrilobular nodules and linear branching opacities on CT and is the most common cause of the "tree-in-bud" pattern. Bacterial organisms are the most common cause of a bronchiolar pattern of disease on CT and viral, parasitic, mycobacterial and fungal organisms are the less common causes.

Aspiration

Bronchiolar changes can be seen on CT after aspiration of infected oralsecretions, other irritant material, or inert material (i.e., barium). The CT findings can include of consolidation, small irregular shadows, and small nodular and linear branching opacities. The distribution of the abnormalities is generally perihilar or bibasilar.

Impaired Host Defenses/Immunologic Deficiencies

Cystic fibrosis
Dyskinetic cilia syndromes

Cigarette Smoking

Respiratory bronchiolitis is a clinicopathologic syndrome that is seen in current heavy cigarette smokers.

Rheumatoid Arthritis and Sjögren's Syndrome

Follicular bronchiolitis is a condition most commonly described in patients with these conditions.

Pullout 3: Approach to Cystic and Cavitary Diseases

Cysts and cavities are commonly encountered abnormalities on chest radiography and chest computed tomography.

Cystic and cavitary lung lesions can be a diagnostic challenge. In such circumstances, distinguishing cysts (wall thickness ⇐4 mm) from cavities (wall thickness > 4 mm or a surrounding infiltrate or mass) and focal or multifocal disease from diffuse involvement facilitates the diagnostic process.

Causes of Focal or Multifocal Cystic and Cavitary Lung Disease

Cystic (wall thickness <4 mm)
Bullae
Blebs
Pneumatoceles
Congenital cystic lesions
Bronchogenic cyst
Congenital adenomatoid malformation
Infections
Coccidioidomycosis
Pneumocystis carinii
Hydatid disease
Traumatic cysts

Cavitary (wall thickness >4 mm or surrounding infiltrate or mass)
Neoplastic
Bronchogenic carcinomas
Metastases
Lymphomas
Infections
Bacteria
Staphylococcus aureus, gram-negative bacteria
pneumococcus, mycobacteria, melioidosis, anaerobes
actinomycosis, nocardiosis
Fungi
Histoplasmosis, coccidioidomycosis, blastomycosis
aspergillosis, mucormycosis, cryptococcosis
P carinii, sporotrichosis
Parasites
Hydatid disease, paragonimiasis, amebiasis
Immunologic
Wegener granulomatosis
Rheumatoid nodule
Thromboembolism or septic embolism
Progressive massive fibrosis (pneumoconiosis)
Bronchiectasis, localized
Congenital lesions
Sequestration
Congenital adenomatoid malformation

Causes of Diffuse Cystic and Cavitary Lung Disease
Pulmonary lymphangioleiomyomatosis
Pulmonary Langerhans cell histiocytosis
Honeycomb lung
Idiopathic pulmonary fibrosis
Connective tissue disease–related pulmonary fibrosis
Asbestosis
Chronic hypersensitivity pneumonitis
Advanced sarcoidosis
Bronchiectasis, diffuse
Metastatic disease (rare)

Pullout 4: Approach to Eosinophilic Lung Disease: A Clinical Overview

The eosinophilic lung diseases are a heterogeneous group of pulmonary disorders characterized by an increase in circulating and tissue eosinophils. Pulmonary eosinophilia can be defined generally as pulmonary infiltrates on radiological imaging together with an increase in the absolute number of eosinophils (> 250/μL) in the peripheral blood.

Classification of Eosinophilic Lung Diseases	**Eosinophilic Lung Diseases Associated with Asthma**
Simple pulmonary eosinophilia	Allergic bronchopulmonary aspergillosis
Chronic eosinophilic pneumonia	Bronchocentric granulomatosis
Acute eosinophilic pneumonia	Chronic eosinophilic pneumonia
Churg-Strauss syndrome	Churg-Strauss syndrome
Idiopathic hypereosinophilic syndrome asthma	
Allergic bronchopulmonary aspergillosis	
Bronchocentric granulomatosis	
Parasitic infections	
Drug reactions	

Parasitic Infections	**Drugs Causing Eosinophilic Lung Disease**
Strongyloides stercoralis	Nitrofurantoin
Ascaris lumbricoides	Phenytoin
Toxocara	Sulfasalazine
Ancylostoma	Ampicillin
Echinococcus	Minocycline
Trichinella spiralis	Methotrexate

Pullout 5: Approach to Parenchymal Lung Diseases

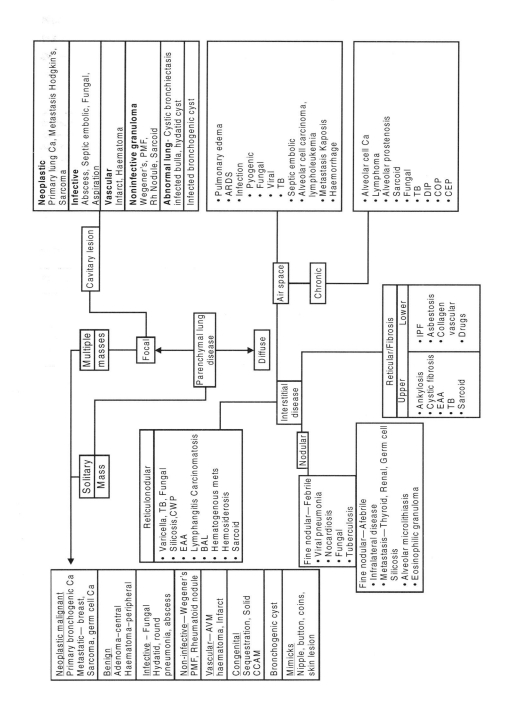

Neoplastic
Primary lung Ca, Metastasis Hodgkin's, Sarcoma
Infective
Abscess, Septic embolic, Fungal, Aspiration
Vascular
Infarct, Haematoma
Noninfective granuloma
Wegener's, PMF, Rh Nodule, Sarcoid
Abnormal lung- Cystic bronchiectasis infected bulla, hydatid cyst
Infected bronchogenic cyst

- Pulmonary edema
- ARDS
- Infection
  - Pyogenic
  - Fungal
  - Viral
  - TB
- Septic embolic
- Alveolar cell carcinoma, lympholeukemia
- Metastasis Kaposis
- Haemorrhage

- Alveolar cell Ca
- Lymphoma
- Alveolar prostenosis
- Sarcoid
- Fungal
- TB
- DIP
- COP
- CEP

Cavitary lesion

Air space

Chronic

Multiple masses

Focal

Parenchymal lung disease

Diffuse

Solitary

Mass

Interstitial disease

Reticular/Fibrosis

Upper	Lower
Ankylosis	IPF
Cystic fibrosis	Asbestosis
EAA	Collagen vascular
TB	Drugs
Sarcoid	

Nodular

Reticulonodular
- Varicella, TB, Fungal
- Silicosis,CWP
- EAA
- Lymphangitis Carcinomatosis
- BAL
- Hematogenous mets
- Hemosiderosis
- Sarcoid

Fine nodular—Febrile
- Viral pneumonia
- Nocardiosis
- Fungal
- Tuberculosis

Fine nodular—Afebrile
- Infralateral disease
- Metastasis—Thyroid, Renal, Germ cell Silicosis
- Alveolar microlithiasis
- Eosinophilic granuloma

Neoplastic malignant
Primary bronchogenic Ca
Metastatic— breast,
Sarcoma, germ cell Ca

Benign
Adenoma-central
Haematoma-peripheral

Infective – Fungal
Hydatid, round
pneumonia, abscess

Non-infective—Wegener's
PMF, Rheumatoid nodule

Vascular—AVM
haematoma, Infarct

Congenital
Sequestration, Solid
CCAM

Bronchogenic cyst

Mimicks
Nipple, button, coins,
skin lesion

Pullout 6: Approach for Reticular Opacity

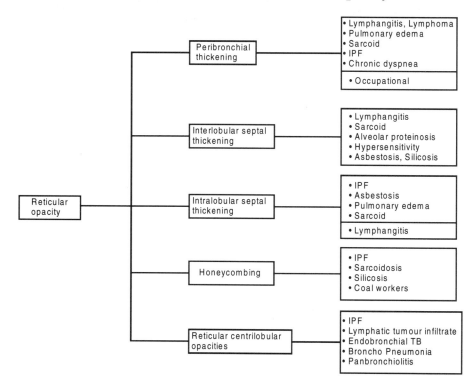

Reticular opacity

- Peribronchial thickening
  - Lymphangitis, Lymphoma
  - Pulmonary edema
  - Sarcoid
  - IPF
  - Chronic dyspnea
  - Occupational

- Interlobular septal thickening
  - Lymphangitis
  - Sarcoid
  - Alveolar proteinosis
  - Hypersensitivity
  - Asbestosis, Silicosis

- Intralobular septal thickening
  - IPF
  - Asbestosis
  - Pulmonary edema
  - Sarcoid
  - Lymphangitis

- Honeycombing
  - IPF
  - Sarcoidosis
  - Silicosis
  - Coal workers

- Reticular centrilobular opacities
  - IPF
  - Lymphatic tumour infiltrate
  - Endobronchial TB
  - Broncho Pneumonia
  - Panbronchiolitis

Pullout 7: Approach for Nodules

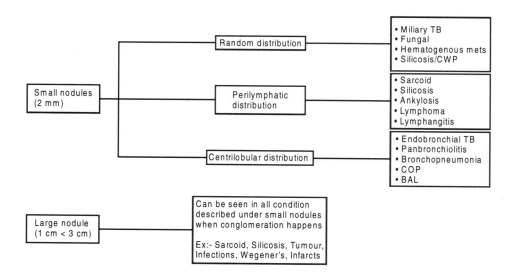

Small nodules (2 mm)

- Random distribution
  - Miliary TB
  - Fungal
  - Hematogenous mets
  - Silicosis/CWP

- Perilymphatic distribution
  - Sarcoid
  - Silicosis
  - Ankylosis
  - Lymphoma
  - Lymphangitis

- Centrilobular distribution
  - Endobronchial TB
  - Panbronchiolitis
  - Bronchopneumonia
  - COP
  - BAL

Large nodule (1 cm < 3 cm)

Can be seen in all condition described under small nodules when conglomeration happens

Ex:- Sarcoid, Silicosis, Tumour, Infections, Wegener's, Infarcts

References

1. HRCT of Lung by Webb, Lippincott Raven.

2. CT and MRI of Whole Body by Haaga, Mosby.

3. CT of the Body by Moss, Saunders.

4. CT and MRI of Chest by Naidich, Lippincott.

5. Imaging of Chest Diseases, by Peterarmstrong, Mosby .

6. Rcna Jan 98, Obstructive Pulmonary Disease.

7. Chest Medicine, June 2002, Tropical Lung Disease.

8. Rcna Sep 91, Imaging of Diffuse Lung Disease.

9. Differential Diagnosis of Disease of the Chest by Fraserpare.

Index

A

Abscess 45
Acinar opacity 47
Acinus 47
Acute intestitial pneumonia 135
Acute necrotizing pneumonia 159
Acute pneumonia 123
Acute respiratory distress syndrome
    extrapulmonary 59
    pulmonary 59
    stages and findings 59
        acute bilateral airspace opacity 60
        air space opacity with fibrotic
            changes 61
        bilaterial multifocal parencymal
            consolidation 60
        CXR 59
        Histopathology 59
Adenocarcinoma 49
    mediastinal lymphadenopathy 49
    solitary peripheral subpleural mass 49
Adhesive atelectasis 138
Aerated acini or lobules 72
Air trapping 50
    differential diagnosis 50
Allergic bronchopulmonary
            aspergillosis 43, 161
Alpha 1 antitrypsin deficiency 91
Alveolar filling diseases
    HRCT findings 48
    time factors 48
Alveolar proteinosis 58
    differential diagnosis 58
Anatomic basis of disease 10
    interstitium 14
    lung parenchymal 11
    normal lung anatomy 10
    secondary pulmonary lobule 14
Approach to
    bronchiolar CT patterns 210
    cystic and cavitary diseases 212
    eosinophilic lung disease 214
    for reticular opacity 216
    ground glass opacity 209
    parencymal lung diseases 215
Architectural distortion 51
    cicatrizial bronchiectatic changes 51
Asbestosis 135
Aspergilloma 52, 160
    differential diagnosis 53
        invasive 53
        semi invasive 53

predisposing pulmonary conditions
        52
Aspiration pneumoniae 27, 45, 62
    CT appearance 63
        with centrolobular nodules 64
        with decreased lung attenuation 64
        with ground-glass attenuation
            and consolidation 64
        with tree-in-bud pattern 63
    diffuse bibasilar alveolar
            consolidation 62
    pathological classification 63
        BOOP 63, 64
        cellular bronchiolitis 63
        constrictive bronchiolitis 63
        respiratory bronchiolitis 63
Asthma 54
Atelectasis 55, 110, 158
    causes 55
        large airway obstruction 55
        small airway obstruction 56
    left lingular resorptive atelectasis 55
    right middle lobe cicatrizial
            atelectasis 55
    types of atelectasis 56
        adhesive atelectasis 56
        cicatrization atelectasis 56
        compressive atelectasis 56
        passive atelectasis 56
Atelectatic pseudotumor 136
Azygous lobe fissure 57
    accessory fissures 57

B

Bacterial lobar/lobular pneumonias 27
Blesovsky syndrome 136
Blunt chest trauma 127
Brochiectasis 95
Bronchial asthma 54
Bronchial atresia 78
    collateral air drift 78
    differential diagnosis 78
    mucous plug 78
    pathogenesis 78
Bronchiectasis 25, 50, 68, 159
    cavitary bronchiectasis 70
    cylindrical bronchiectasis 68
    cystic bronchiectasis 68
    predisposing condition 70
        kartagener's syndrome 69
        middle lobe syndrome 69

Mounier-Kuhn syndrome 69
Swyer-James syndrome 69
Williams-Campbell syndrome 69
yellow-nail syndrome 69
young's syndrome 69
varicose bronchiestasis 69
Bronchiectatic cyst 85
Bronchiolectasis 65
Bronchiolitis obliterans organizing
            pneumonia 74
    bilateral multisegmental peripheral
            consolidations 74
    BOOP pathology 74
    clinical features 75
    granulation tissue polyps 74
Broncho alveolar carcinoma 72, 73
    bilateral confluent alveolar opacity 73
    bilateral multifocal parenchymal
            lobar consolidation 73
Bronchogenic cyst 76
    bronchopulmonary foregut
            malformations 77
    clinical manifestations 76
    marginated hypodense lesion 76
    pathophysiology 76
Broncholithiasis 66
    causes 66
    CT findings 66
        calcified nodes 66
        endobronchial calcifications 66
    symptoms 66
Bronchopleural fistula 67
    CT findings 67
        features of empyema 67
        peripheral bronchopleural fistula
            67
Bronchostenosis 159
Bubble lucencies 72
Bulla 71
    classification 71
    CT findings 71
    differential diagnosis 71
Bullae and blebs 25

C

Calcified peribronchial nodes 66
Cavitating lung carcinoma 46
Cavitation 158
Cavitatory nodules 25
Cavity 79
    adjacent parenchymal nodular
            opacities 79

marginated cavitary lesions 79
marginated lucent parenchymal
        zones 79
mechanism 79
pulmonary lucency 79
Central bronchiectasis 44
Centrilobular abnormalities 21
Chronic eosinophilic pneumonia 86
    clinical features of 86
        acute eosinophilic 86
        chronic eosinophilic 86
        Loffler's syndrome 86
        tropical eosinophilia 86
    CT findings 86
Cicatricial ectasia 95
Cicatricial fibrosis 92
Collagen vascular disease 26, 29, 135
Compensatory hyperinflation 84
    increase in right lung volume 84
    substernal herniation 84
Compression atelectasis 87
Compressive atelectasis 153
Concept of
    cortical lung 15
    medullary lung 15
Congenital cystic adenomatoid
        malformation 88
    coalescent cystic lesion 88
Congenital lobar emphysema 87
    hyperinflation of right middle lobe 87
    passive atelectasis of the lower lobe 87
Conglomerate fibrosis 95
Conglomerate mass 80
    adjacent parenchymal cicatrizial
        changes 80
    bilateral upper zone parenchymal
        mass lesion 80
    in sarcoidosis 80
    pneumoconiosis 80
Consolidation 23, 60, 81, 158, 159
    four stages 81
    infective pneumonia 81
        expected time for resolution 82
        pattern of involvement 82
    with air bronchogram 81
CRESR syndrome 143
Cyst 83
    differential diagnosis 83
    honeycombing with cyst formation 83
    multiple lucent spaces with
        conglomeration 83
Cystic bronchiectatic changes 110
Cystic fibrosis 85

D

Desquamative interstitial pneumonia 29,
        135
Diffuse alveolar damage 29

Diffuse lung diseases 33
Drug-induced lung disease 89, 135
    bilateral multifocal alveolar opacity 89
    imaging by different group of drugs
        89
    alveolar hemorrhage 90
    drug-induced SLE 90
    interstitial inflammation 89
    noncardiogenic pulmonary
        edema 90
    pulmonary infiltrates with
        eosinophilia 90
Dysplasia 87

E

Embolism/infarction 93
    CT findings 93
        linear bands and atelectasis 93
        lung attenuation 93
        pleural effusion 93
        pleural parenchymal
            consolidation 93
        wedge shaped 93
Emphysema 24, 91
    centrilobular emphysema 91
    irregular emphysema 92
    panacinar emphysema 91
    paraseptal emphysema 92
Empyema 67
End-stage lung 95
Endobronchial obstruction 94
    axial CECT section at carinal 94
    classification 94
        extrinsic lesion 94
        metastasis 94
        neoplasm 94
        non-neoplastic lesions 94
    virtual bronchoscopy images 94
Endobronchial spread 159
Eosinophilic pneumonia 29
Ewings tumor 96
    differential diagnosis 96
    expansile osteolytic lesion of 8th rib
        96
    soft tissue component of rib lesion 96
    SSD of ribs 96
Extrinsic allergic alveolitis 101

F

FDG-PET imaging 32
Fibrosing allergic alveolitis 26
Fibrosis 135
Fibrotic disease 92, 139
Fibrotic lung disease 19
Fissural fluid 98
    fluid within the fissures 98
Focal abnormality 31

imaging features 31
    biological activity 32
    cavitation 32
    contrast enhancement 32
    feeding vessel sign 32
    halosign 32
    lesion growth 31
    lesion size 31
    lesion texture 31
    margins 31
    positive bronchus sign 32
associated radiological findings 38
    cavities 33
    distribution 38
    radiological pattern 34
        chronic lung scarring 37
        consolidation 35
        cystic air spaces 35
        ground glass opacities 37
        linear or reticular opacities 35
        small nodules 35
        thickened interlobular septa 37
    solitary masses and nodules 33
    tempo of disease 34
Focal lung disease 30
Focal lung lesion 31
Folded lung syndrome 136
Fungal abscess 97
    axial CT 97
        invasive aspergillosis 97
        mucormycosis 97
Fungal pneumonias 97

G

Goodpasture's syndrome 27, 103
Ground glass opacities 23
Ground glass opacity 99
    axial CT 99
        desquamative alveolitis 99
        hemorrhage 99
    causes of 99
        diffuse pattern of GGO 99
        focal pattern of GGO 99

H

Helical atelectasis 136
Hemosiderin 103
Hemosiderin-laden macrophages 103
High attenuation mucus plug 44
High-resolution CT (HRCT) 3
    artifacts on HRCT 4
    collimation 3
    CT for chest survey 6
    expiratory scan 7
    field of view 4
    image photography 4
    indication 3

matrix size 4
motion artifacts 5
prone scan 7
reconstruction algorithm 3
scan protocols 5
scan technique 3
scan time 3
star artifacts 5
streak artifacts 4
thoracic evaluation for hemoptysis 6
window setting 4
Hilar lymphadenopathy 139, 158
Hilar retraction 95
HIV associated pneumoniae 129
Honeycomb lung 29
Honeycombing 21, 24, 100
    bilateral subpleural conglomerate
        cysts 100
    CT findings with associated
        pathology 100
Honeycombing with a fibrotic pattern 95
Horner's syndrome 118
HRCT findings of lung disease 19
    cystic abnormalities 24
    decreased lung opacities 24
    increased lung opacities 23
    linear and reticular opacities 19
    nodules and nodular opacities 21
Hydropneumothorax 124
Hypercapnia 28
Hyperlucent hemithorax 105
Hypersensitive pneumonitis 101
    acute axial CT lung 102
    chronic axial CT 102
    subacute axial CT 101
Hypoxemia 28, 29

I

Idiopathic pneumonias 135
Idiopathic pulmonary fibrosis 135
Idiopathic pulmonary hemosiderosis 27
Interface sign 19
Interlobular septal thickening 20, 146
Interstitial lung disease 25
Intralobular interstitial thickening 20
Irregular bronchiectasis 155

K

Kerley's B lines 146
Koch's lesion 157
Kochs diseases 156

L

Large nodules 22
Lobar atelectasis 159

Loeffler's syndrome 27
Lung calcification 23
Lung cysts 24
Lung neoplasm 144
Lung volume 116
Lymphadenopathy 38, 159
Lymphangioleiomyomatosis 106
    bilateral diffuse discrete thin walled
        cysts 106
    CT findings 106
    differential diagnosis 106
Lymphangitic carcinomatosis 107
    bilateral nodular septal thickening 107
    metastasis due to carcinoma
        stomach 107
Lymphangitic metastases 142

M

Mendelson syndrome 62
Mesothelioma 111
    CT findings 111
    differential diagnosis 111
    pathophysiology 111
Middle lobe syndrome 110
    complication 110
    CT findings 110
    etiology 110
Miliary disease 159
Miliary nodules 108
Miliary pattern 108
    differential diagnosis and algorithm
        axial HRCT punctate nodules 108
Miliary tuberculosis 108, 158
Mitotic lung lesion 49
Mosaic perfusion 109
    CT findings 109
        airway disease 109
        primary vascular disease 109
    mosaic pattern 109
Mucoid impaction 50
Mucus plugs 50

N

Necrotizing aspergillosis 52
Necrotizing granuloma 164
Necrotizing pneumonitis 46
Neoplasia 112
    bronchogenic carcinoma 112
    rare primary neoplasms 114
        adenoid cystic carcinoma 114
        bronchial adenomas 114
        mucoepidermoid carcinoma 114
    staging 113
        adenocarcinoma 113
        bronchioalveolar 113
        lare cell Ca 114
        pancoast's tumor 114

small cell Ca 114
squamous cell Ca 113
Nodular opacity 30
Nodules 115, 159
    multiple large nodules 115
    well marginated nodules 115
Nonspecific interstitial pneumonia 135
Normal CT lung anatomy 7

O

Obstructive hyperinflation
    calcified retrocarnial lymph node
        116
    mechanism 116
Osler-Weber-Rendu diseases 131

P

Pancoast syndrome 118
Pancoast tumor 118
    osteolytic lesion with adjacent soft
        tissue lesion 118
    soft tissue density lesion with
        cavitary changes 118
Paraneoplastic syndrome 112
Parenchymal band 20
Parenchymal band-linear 117
    differential diagnosis 117
    HRCT findings 117
Parenchymal scars 49
Parenchymatous lung disease 27
    interstitial pattern 28
    intra-alveolar pattern 27
    intra-alveolar/interstitial pattern 29
    normal pattern 27
Partial airway obstruction 50
Partial bronchial obstruction 116
Pectoralis major muscle 133
Peribronchovascular interstitial
        thickening 19
Pleural calcification 120
Pleural deposits 126
    axial CT chest in mediastinal
        window 126
    causes 126
Pleural disease 159
Pleural effusion 122, 158, 159
    fissural fluid 122
    large left pleural effusion 122
    large pleural effusion, passive
        atelectasis and fissural fluid
        122
    passive atelectasis 122
Pleural effusion thickening 38
Pleural thickening 121
    causes 121
    CT findings 121

diffuse thickening of parietal pleural
121
focal pleural deposit 121
Pleuroma 136
Pneumatocele 25, 123
causes 123
CT findings 123
cystic space in the left lingua 123
pathogenesis 123
Pneumocystis carinii pneumonia 129
HRCT findings 129
infections associated with AIDS 129
Pneumothorax 124
air in the right pleural space 124
classification 124
left lowerlobe patchy alveolar
opacity 125
primary spontaneous pneumothorax
125
secondary spontaneous
pneumothorax 124
Poland syndrome 133
chest wall with absence of pectoralis
major muscle 133
Primary-Mounier-Kuhn syndrome 154
Pulmonary alveolar proteinosis 27
Pulmonary AV malformation 131
complications 131
CT demonstrates 131
location 131
types 131
vascular causes of 131
atriovenous malformation 131
pulmonary artery aneurysm 132
pulmonary varix 132
Pulmonary contusion 127
Pulmonary edema 86, 128
bilateral confluent air space opacity 128
radiological pattern for 128
capillary injury 128
cardiogenic 128
radiological sign 128
renal 128
Pulmonary eosinophilia 27
Pulmonary hemorrhage 103
acute pulmonary hemorrhage 103
causes of hemoptysis 104
causes of intra alveolar hemorrhage
104
differential diagnosis 103
diffuse pulmonary hemorrhage 103
Pulmonary laceration 130
ovoid or elliptical lucencies with air-
fluid 130
Purulent liquefaction necrosis 45

R

Radiation pneumonitis 135, 138
bilateral paramediastinal ground
glass attenuation 138

Rasmussen's aneurysm 134, 160
CT findings 134
differential diagnosis 134
Raynaud's phenomenon 143
Resorption atelectasis 94, 138
Respiratory distress syndrome 29
Reticular pattern 135
bilateral peripheral reticular
opacities honeycombing 135
Rheumatoid lung 137
high-resolution CT 137
bronchiolectasis 137
fibrosis 137
ground-glass opacity 137
honeycombing 137
interlobular septal thickening 137
large nodular opacities 137
pleural thickening effusion 137
small centrilobular nodules 137
traction bronchiectasis 137
Round atelectasis 136
lung window with subpleural lesion
136
pathogenesis 136

S

Sarcoid 92
Sarcoidosis 141, 29, 38
CT findings 141
differential diagnosis 142
staging of sarcoid 141
Secondaries 144
calcifying metastases 145
cavitating metastases 145
common primaries 144
diagnosis of primary tumor 144
endobronchial metastases 145
hemorrhage metastases 145
Secondary tracheomegaly 95
Septal thickening 146
Sequestration 152
extralobar sequestration (ELS) 152
intralobar sequestration (ILS) 152
pulmonary venous drainage 152
Shrinking pleuritis with atelectasis
136
Signs in thoracic CT 166
air bronchogram sign 166
air crescent sign 167
CT angiogram sign 174
drowned lung sign 168
fallen lung sign 169
gloved finger sign 170
golden's sign 171
halo sign 172
hampton's hump sign 173
luftsichel sign 178
signet-ring sign 175

split pleura sign 176
westermark sign 177
Silico tuberculosis 139
Silicosis 38, 80, 139
bilateral multiple centrilobular
nodules 139
Small nodules 21
Solitary Pulmonary Nodule 148
appearance of SPN on CT scanning
150
differential diagnosis 148
factors of malignant vs benign SPN 151
Spontaneous pneumothorax 92
Subpleural bullae 92
Subpleural interstitial thickening 20
Subpleural lines 21, 147
Superior pulmonary sulcus tumor 118
Suppurative necrosis 45
Swyer-James syndrome 64, 105
Systemic sclerosis (scleroderma) 143
Systemic vasculitides 27

T

Tension pneumothorax 87
Thoracentesis 122
Three dimensional rendering
techniques 162
imaging techniques 162
three-dimensional intensitty
projection 162
three-dimensional shaded surface
display 162
two-dimensional multiplanar
reconstruction 162
volume rendering 162
Tracheomegaly 154
Traction bronchiectasis 155
Traction ectactic changes 155
Traction ectasia 155
Transbronchial spread 156
Tree-in-BUD 161
Tuberculosis 157
clinical 158
complications 160
postprimary tuberculosis 159
primary tuberculosis 158
radiologic findings 159
hematogenous dissemination 157
pathogenesis 157

U

Useful hints for chest imaging 179
diffuse interstitial disease 181
extrapulmonary physical findings
182
filling pattern on chest
radiograph 184

disease characterized by
cystic abnormalities 195
decreased lung opacity 195
emphysema and bronchiectasis 195
HRCT patterns in interstitial lung disease 199
increased parenchymal opacification 192
linear and reticular opacities 184
nodular and reticulonodular opacity 188

guidelines to evaluate 200
diffuse lung diseases 200
diffuse parenchymal lung disease 201
infections 203
diagnostic tests for opportunistic infections 203
infectious pulmonary complications of AIDS 205
noninfectious pulmonary complications of AIDS 205

lower lobe 181
upper lobe 181
Usual interstitial pneumonia 135

W

Wegener's granuloma 46, 164
clinical presentation 164
airway involvement 164
bilateral reticulo-nodular opacities 164
lab parameters 164